Bulimia
A Guide to Recovery
Fifth Edition

Lindsey Hall
and
Leigh Cohn

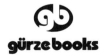

gürze books

Bulimia: A Guide to Recovery
Fifth Edition

© 1999 by Lindsey Hall & Leigh Cohn

Gürze Books
P.O. Box 2238
Carlsbad, CA 92018
(760) 434-7533
www.gurze.com

Cover design by Abacus Graphics, Oceanside, CA
Original Fabric art by Dorothy Turk

Publishing History:
Copyright ©1999, this Fifth Edition has been expanded and is fully revised and updated based on the following, previously published editions: Bulimia: A Guide to Recovery "Revised Edition" (Gürze Books, 1992); Eating Without Fear (Bantam Books, 1990); Bulimia: A Guide to Recovery (Gürze Books, 1986); Set of three booklets (Gürze Books, 1980-83).

Library of Congress
Cataloging-in-Publication Data
Hall, Lindsey, 1949-
    Bulimia: a guide to recovery.
    Includes index.
1. Bulimia.   2. Eating disorders   3. Psychotherapy   4. Self-care, health
I. Cohn, Leigh.   II. Title.
ISBN 0-936077-31-X   86-045375

NOTE:
The authors and publisher of this book intend for this publication to provide accurate information. It is sold with the understanding that it is meant to complement, not substitute for, professional medical and/or psychological services.

6 8 0 9 7

This book is due for return on or before the last date shown below.

BOOKS BY LINDSEY HALL & LEIGH COHN

(Published by Gürze Books unless noted)

Anorexia Nervosa: A Guide to Recovery, 1998
by Lindsey Hall & Monika Ostroff

Bulimia: A Guide to Recovery—Fifth Edition, 1999

Dear Kids of Alcoholics, 1988

*Dear Kids of Alcoholics Guidebook
for Counselors, Educators & Parents,* 1988

Eating Disorders: A Reference Sourcebook, 1999
by Raymond Lemberg with Leigh Cohn (Oryx Press)

*Full Lives: Women Who Have Freed Themselves from
Food and Weight Obsession,* 1993 by Lindsey Hall

*Making Weight: Men's Conflicts with Food, Weight, Shape &
Appearance,* 2000 by ArnoldAndersen, M.D., Leigh Cohn,
M.A.T., and Thomas Holbrook, M.D.

*Recoveries: True Stories of People who Conquered
Addictions and Compulsions,* 1987 (out of print)

Self-Esteem: Tools for Recovery, 1990

Sexual Abuse and Eating Disorders: A Clinical Overview,
1996 by Mark Schwartz & Leigh Cohn (Brunner/Mazel)

*Let us all
love and respect
each other
and ourselves.*

Table of Contents

Chapter 2. Eat Without Fear: A True Story of the Binge-Purge Syndrome

PART II. Overcoming Bulimia

Chapter 3. How to Start

Chapter 4. Get Support! 117

Chapter 5. What Has Worked for Many 133

Introduction

I am wide awake and immediately out of bed. I think back to the night before when I made a new list of what I wanted to get done and how I wanted to be. My husband is not far behind me on his way into the bathroom to get ready for work. Maybe I can sneak onto the scale before he notices me. I am already in my private world. I am overjoyed when the scale says that I stayed the same weight as I was the night before, and I can feel that slightly hungry feeling. Maybe IT will stop today, maybe today everything will change. What were the projects I wanted to do?

We eat the same breakfast, except that I take no butter on my toast, no cream in my coffee and never take seconds (until he gets out the door). Today I am going to be really good, which means eating certain predetermined portions of food and not taking one more bite than I think I am allowed. I am careful to see that I don't take more than he does. I can feel the tension building. I wish he'd hurry up and leave so I can get going!

As soon as he shuts the door, I try to involve myself with one of the myriad of responsibilities on my list. But I hate them all! I just want to crawl into a hole. I don't want to do anything. I'd rather eat. I am alone, I am nervous, I am no good, I always do every-

thing wrong anyway. I am not in control, I can't make it through the day, I know it. It has been the same for so long.

I remember the starchy cereal I ate for breakfast. I am into the bathroom and onto the scale. It measures the same, BUT I DON'T WANT TO STAY THE SAME! I want to be thinner! I look in the mirror. I think my thighs are ugly and deformed looking. I see a lumpy, clumsy, pear-shaped wimp. I feel frustrated, trapped in this body, and I don't know what to do about it.

I float to the refrigerator knowing exactly what is inside. I begin with last night's brownies. I always begin with the sweets. At first I try to make it look like nothing is missing, but my appetite is huge and I resolve to make another batch of brownies to replace the one I'm devouring. I know there is half of a bag of cookies in the trash, thrown out the night before, and I dig them out and polish them off. I drink some milk so my vomiting will be smoother. I like the full feeling I get after downing a big glass. I get out six pieces of bread and toast one side in the broiler, turn them over and cover them with butter and put them under the broiler again till they are bubbling. I take all six pieces on a plate to the television and go back for a bowl of cereal and a banana. Before the last toast is finished, I am already preparing the next batch of six more pieces. I might have another brownie or five from the new batch, and a couple large bowlfuls of ice cream, yogurt, or cottage cheese. My stomach is stretched into a huge ball below my ribcage. I know I'll have to go into the bathroom soon, but I want to postpone it. I am in never-never land. I am waiting, feeling the pressure, pacing the floor in and out of rooms. Time is passing. Time is passing. It is almost time.

I wander aimlessly through the living room and kitchen one more time, tidying, making the whole house neat and put back together. Finally, I make the turn into the bathroom. I brace my feet, pull my hair back and stick my finger down my throat, stroking twice. I get up a huge gush of food. Three times, four and another stream of partially-digested food. I can see everything come back. I am glad to see those brownies because they are SO fattening. The rhythm of the emptying is broken and my head is beginning to hurt. I stand up feeling dizzy, empty and weak. The whole episode has taken about an hour.

For nine years, I binged and vomited up to five times daily. Although there were a few days without a binge, the thoughts were always there, even in my dreams. It was painful and frightening. No one knew about my bulimia, because I kept it safely hidden behind a facade of competence, happiness, and average body weight. When my health and marriage began to fail, however, a series of coincidences brought me face to face with recovery, and I soon became devoted to freeing myself from my obsession with food.

I worked hard and willingly, and underwent an amazing transformation. As the bulimic thoughts and behavior subsided, I was able to see how it had served me all those years. It was an effective tool for emotional, physical, and spiritual survival when I knew no other. It had been a friend, a lover, a hiding place, a voice, a quest for meaning and love. It was a way to cope with growing up in a frightening and uncertain world. But what had started as an innocent diet became a monster which threatened to devour my entire life.

My healing was not an overnight thing. I spent a year-and-a-half gradually letting go of the bulimic behavior, examining every binge for its meaning and purpose. After another year or so, I was able to eat more than just my "safe" foods, and eventually, I became comfortable living in my body, instead of feeling trapped. I also stopped judging other people's bodies, no matter what their shape or size—something that is very difficult to do in a culture that promotes weight prejudice.

One of the most profound revelations I had in recovery was that I didn't know who I was or would be without the bulimia. So, in order to know myself at a deeper level, I purposefully shifted my focus from what I looked like on the outside to what I thought and felt on the inside. I did this through meditation, journal and letter writing, long walks, and deep conversations. I discovered that I was a good and loving person with ups and downs like everyone else, and once I made the connection to this inner life, everything began to change. I am now healthy, happy, and completely free from bulimia, and have been for over twenty years.

In 1980 when my husband, Leigh Cohn, and I wrote my story in a booklet titled, *Eat Without Fear,* there were no other publications available solely on bulimia. The response was tremendous! This little booklet was inspiring and motivated many others who were trying to quit; and, as we learned more about the binge-purge syndrome, we realized there was more to say.

Over the next few years, we gave many talks around the country, and I became the first person to share her story of bulimia on national television. We wrote several books, including *BULIMIA: A Guide to Recovery*, of which there are now more than 100,000 copies in print in various forms. We also created a small publishing company specializing in books on eating disorders written by a variety of respected authors. This expanded and updated version of *BULIMIA: A Guide to Recovery* is the result of our combined personal experience serving the entire eating disorders community—the individuals suffering from these disorders, their loved ones, therapists, educators, and researchers—for over twenty years.

This book is divided into two main parts. The first, "Understanding Bulimia," answers questions often asked, and includes my own story, *Eat Without Fear*. The second section, "Overcoming Bulimia," offers motivation, support, inspiration, specific recovery suggestions, things to do instead of bingeing, and advice for loved-ones. "A Three-Week Program to Stop Bingeing" is included here. This is not intended to be a quick cure, but rather an initial experience of self-love to motivate readers to further pursue their recovery. Written in a personal, instructive, inspirational tone, the program includes day-by-day activities, exercises, and written assignments. The instructions are direct and specific, but demand attention and dedication. This is followed by "A Guide for Support Groups" which includes six agendas and activities for bulimia groups. We have also included resources for further information.

Throughout the book are quotes in italics. Many are from recovered and recovering bulimics and eating disorders therapists who responded to two questionnaires we mailed out in 1983 and 1991. Overall, we received 392 honest and personal impressions on subjects such as: recovering from eating disorders, therapy options, the role of family and friends, and helpful activities in overcoming all kinds of destructive eating. Also, in this fifth edition are quotes from the many letters we've received from readers who have wanted to share their experiences of recovery, or thank us for our support.

The individuals who offer their quotes come from diverse backgrounds; the only apparent element common to all of them is that they have an understanding of bulimia because of their direct experiences with it. They generously shared their insight with us, and we are passing it along to you.

Much of this book is addressed to "you," readers with bulimia; and, since most bulimics are women, we use feminine pronouns. However, the information and practical self-help tools are equally useful for men. Additionally, although "I" am the "speaker," Leigh equally contributed to the writing, ideas, and publishing of this effort, and sometimes "we" both speak in the text.

For over twenty years, Leigh and I have worked full-time on eating disorders education and publications. We have become well-known in this field, work with most of the national eating disorders organizations, attend national and international conferences, and continue to write and speak about recovery. Our company, Gürze Books has published more than 25 titles and is best-known for the *Gürze Eating Disorders Resource Catalogue*, which is a comprehensive selection of books and tapes compiled from various sources. We also publish the *Eating Disorders Review*, a newsletter for clinicians; and, our website (www.bulimia.com) is a much-travelled gateway to eating disorders information.

When I first wrote *Eat Without Fear* in 1980, I did so as a way to bring closure to my recovery from bulimia. I did not expect or intend to become more involved with this subject. However, sharing my experience has remained an integral part of my life, because of the effect it has had on others.

PART ONE

Understanding Bulimia

CHAPTER 1

Questions Most Often Asked About Bulimia

What is bulimia?

Bulimia is an obsession with food and weight characterized by repeated overeating binges followed by compensatory behavior, such as forced vomiting or excessive exercise. For an epidemic number of women and men, bulimia is a secret addiction that dominates their thoughts, undercuts their self-esteem, and threatens their lives. The symptoms are described by the Egyptians and in the Hebrew Talmud; and bulimia (Greek for "ox-hunger") was widely practiced during Greek and Roman times. In the later half of the twentieth century, though, eating disorders, and particularly bulimia, have been identified as widespread cultural phenomena. Bulimia is also termed bulimia nervosa and bulimarexia.

In 1980, the American Psychiatric Association formally recognized bulimia. In its fourth edition, the Diagnostic and Statistical Manual of Mental Disorders (APA, 1994) lists the following criteria that an individual must meet to be diagnosed:

A. Recurrent episodes of binge eating, with an episode characterized by (1) eating in a discrete period of time, usually less than two hours, an amount of food that is significantly larger than most people would eat during a similar period of time and under similar circumstances; and, (2) a sense of lack of control over eating during the episode, such as a feeling that one cannot stop eating.

B. Recurrent inappropriate compensatory behavior in order to prevent weight gain, such as self-induced vomiting, misuse of laxatives, diuretics, or enemas (purging type); or, through fasting or excessive exercise (nonpurging type).

C. These behaviors occur at least twice a week for at least three months.

D. Self-evaluation is unduly influenced by body shape and weight.

E. The behavior does not only occur during episodes of anorexia nervosa.

The above list was created to help clinicians diagnose and treat this complex disorder. However, many individuals, termed "subclinical," fulfill only some of the criteria. These cases are also life-damaging and need to be taken seriously.

Although the overt symptoms of bulimia revolve around food behaviors and a fear of gaining weight, bulimia is actually a way to cope with personal distress and emotional pain. Eating binges take time and focus away from more disturbing issues, and purges are an effective way to regain the control and feelings of safety lost during the binge. Also, while bulimic behavior may have started as a seemingly-innocent way to lose weight, the cycle of bingeing and purging usually becomes an addictive escape from all kinds of other problems.

Most individuals with bulimia are extremely secretive about their behavior, sometimes going to great lengths to maintain the appearance of normal eating around other people. They are ashamed of their behavior and what it has done to their lives. Many describe feeling like two people—one who wants to give it up and be healthy, and another who constantly sabotages. Lying and sneaking are common traits. Many people describe stealing food that they know belongs to other people or digging through the trash during particularly desperate episodes.

Although a typical binge represents a large quantity of food, usually between 1500 and 3000 calories and primarily high carbohydrates, a binge is uniquely defined by the person doing it. Even a "normal" meal might feel like "too much" to someone who is terrified of getting fat.

Binges can be triggered in a number of ways: by higher numbers on a scale, eating something that is normally forbidden or taking one bite more than allowed, difficult feelings, a traumatic event, or something as innocuous as thinking about food. Many people describe their feelings during binges as completely out of control, driven by a desperate desire to feel even a little bit better. While they might feel ugly, unworthy, hopeless, and helpless before and during a binge/purge episode, after, they might feel a mix of control, shame, relief, disgust, dizziness, exhaustion, and resolution. Part of the cycle often includes the promise that each time will be the last.

It is difficult to say how many people have bulimia. Statistics may not truly reflect the total numbers because, as we said, bulimics generally hide their behavior. In fact, one study showed that college students answered questionnaires more truthfully when told to put a dab of their saliva on the survey paper, because they believed it could be chemically analyzed to determine if they were bulimic!

Of the research done on the prevalence of eating disorders, the most reliable statistics indicate that about 5% of college-aged women meet the strict clinical criteria for bulimia. However, some studies offer much higher numbers. A recent one of female high school and college students reported that 15% met the criteria for bulimia (Cavanaugh, 1999), and some experts suggest that as many as one of every three women have engaged in some bulimic behavior. Men account for at least 10% of cases, although, this number has seemed to increase in recent years. There is also evidence that—unlike anorexia nervosa, which has remained fairly constant in the past few decades—the incidence of bulimia rose significantly in the early 1980's (Russell, 1997). Whatever the actual figures, a significant number of both women and men are engaging in this self-destructive behavior.

Why do people become bulimic?

There is no easy answer to this question. Just as the life of every individual is unique, so are the reasons why they become bulimic and the paths they must take to overcome it.

Bulimia is generally considered to be a psychological and emotional disorder, which sometimes coexists with other psychiatric disorders, such as depression or obsessive compulsive disorder. Some studies show that bulimia is related to major affective disorder, (Johnson, 1987) and therefore influenced by heredity and chemical imbalances in the body. (See "Can medication help in recovery?" in this chapter.) In some cases, therefore, medication can alleviate the binge-purge behavior or the blanket of depression, making psychotherapy and other avenues for recovery more effective. Other studies have linked lowered brain serotonin function to bulimia (Kaye, 1999). However, the underlying reasons most people give for their eating disorder are a complex mix of low self-esteem, childhood conflicts, and cultural pressures.

In general, people become addicted to substances and behaviors to avoid painful feelings—past as well as present. Some of these feelings have their origins in childhood, such as feeling unloved and unlovable, ashamed, afraid, or incompetent. Others come from the pressure to conform or to be accepted by peers. Most devastating of all are the feelings associated with low self-esteem—that we have no worth, that our lives have no value or purpose, and that we will never be fulfilled or happy.

Paradoxically, an eating disorder in the early stages can raise self-esteem when it provides someone with a sense of success—in this case by achieving the cultural ideal of thinness. Indeed, many individuals turn to purging when they have failed at a diet and fear that there is no other way for them to lose weight. However, once the bingeing and purging cycle begins, the resulting metabolic imbalances and habitual escape become an ever-deepening pit, eventually eroding any initial sense of self-worth and control. It is important for those who are reading this book to remember that the rewards for thinness are only implied, and although diets and a thinner body promise a happier life, they don't deliver!

The question remains as to why bulimia is the chosen escape, and there appear to be similarities in the backgrounds, personalities and experiences of eating disordered individuals which will help clarify this. All of these characteristics will not apply to everyone, but certainly some will.

Most bulimics come from families in which the emotional, physical, or spiritual needs of family members are not met in some way. In some of these households, feelings are not verbally expressed and communication skills are lacking. There may be a history of depression, alcoholism, drug abuse, or eating disorders; and, the child might unconsciously recognize that escape is an appropriate thing to do. In this context, food becomes a "good" drug, something which does not have the negative connotations of alcohol or drug abuse.

Bulimics are often considered "ideal" children, and will go out of their way to be "people pleasers." They present an acceptable facade—seeming outgoing, confident, and independent—while anxious feelings bubble underneath. They may be valued for not needing to be nurtured, for taking care of themselves, and for growing up early. Bulimia is a way of expressing what cannot be said directly in words, in this case something like, "I want to be taken care of," or "Will you love me as I am?"

Sometimes, people use bulimia to postpone growing up. The child who has looked to others for validation and feelings of self-worth and who has assumed a "perfect little girl" role because it works at home may experience tremendous fear at having to trust herself and face the outside world alone. This insecurity is sometimes unconsciously reinforced by parents who also do not want to let go.

Often parents and children fall into roles that limit the relationships and personal growth within the family. Mothers may reinforce the idea that it is important for women to be thin. Fathers may be relegated to the role of economic provider and disciplinarian rather than taking part in a son's or daughter's emotional life. Girls, in particular, can develop insecurities about their appearance, competence, and ability to be loved if they are not valued for their own unique strengths. In a society where roles for women are changing, strong relationships with parents of both sexes based on the child's uniqueness will give him or her the confidence and ability to make smart decisions and negotiate healthy relationships in the future.

Bulimics tend to be overly judgmental of themselves and others, have difficulty expressing emotions through language, fear criticism, avoid disagreements, and have low self-esteem—all traits which make having relationships with others difficult. In fact, many people in our survey of 392 recovered and recovering bulimics indicated that they were uncomfortable with intimate relationships, and that bulimia was their predictable, reliable, unquestioning ally. Many had been sexually or emotionally abused as children and had difficulty trusting others. The bulimic rituals and thoughts protected them from what might be rejection, abandonment, or other potential pain. The bulimia had become the only relationship, albeit an empty one, which also prevented them from experiencing deep love—described on one woman's survey as "The Great Filler."

The bulimics from our survey identified various causes for their disorder. Many remembered specific reasons for their initial binges, as well as how the behavior subsequently served them. Few women thought it would become addictive. In addition to the original causes which still existed, they were faced with guilt, secrecy, physical side-effects, and an increasing number of reasons to want to escape. Frequently mentioned were: boredom, the influences of media and culture, family dynamics, mental "numbness," the irresistible taste of food, pressure to lose weight, the "high" experienced after purging, overwhelming bouts of anxiety, the release of physical and sexual tension.

Most bulimics have been preoccupied with eating and diet for years, but the initial binge-purge episodes might be triggered by specific events, such as: traumatic change (graduation, moving away from home, marriage, death of a loved one, etc.), unresolved grief, career changes, a failed diet, and rejection by a lover or wished-for lover. These survey comments were among the several specific reasons offered for starting the bulimic behavior:

I started because I was rejected by a boy at age 15. I thought the only main thing wrong with me was my weight.

I developed my eating disorder the night before my first college finals. My father had passed away a month earlier, and I was nervous about my tests and about returning home and having him not be there.

I never thought about trying it until I read about it.

I started throwing up during my fourth month of pregnancy, when I could not handle my changing body and dieting away the calories became impossible.

One of my friends showed me how to do it when we were at junior high. Looking back, she didn't do me any favors!

No matter what the underlying reasons, bulimia "works" on many different levels. Binge-eating provides instant relief. It replaces all other actions, thoughts, and emotions. The mind ceases to dwell on anything but food and how to get it down. Feelings are on hold. Even vomiting can be pleasurable when it is the most intimate contact we allow with our own bodies. When the whole binge-purge episode is over, for a brief moment, the bulimic regains control. No longer feeling guilty for having eaten so many calories, she is drained, relaxed, and high.

Since bulimia is falsely perceived as less dangerous than alcoholism or drug abuse, it is especially insidious and captivating. Food is always available for a "fix," and eating in public, even if on the run, is accepted and not unusual. Also, nothing gives a bulimic away, because her weight usually appears close to normal. Food gives life, heals, nurtures, and means love. The safety, relief, availability, pleasure, and companionship represented by food appear to outweigh any immediate drawbacks. Bulimia becomes a short-term solution for pain, which in the long term can be devastating.

Hopefully, everyone reading this book now understands that an eating disorder is a painful, exhausting illness. Anyone suffering through it deserves tremendous compassion and empathy. Judging them as wasteful, self-centered, vain or spoiled, invalidates that person's feelings, ignores underlying issues, and increases the individual's shame. Remember, an eating disorder is not just about food.

Why are bulimics mainly women?

In the most simple terms, we live in a society which is fundamentally unsatisfying to an enormous number of women, and eating disorders are a symbol of this inner emptiness. Many of our institutions, corporations, systems and roles are set up in a male-oriented, hierarchical structure. This type of environment, which favors independence and competition, alienates those women who feel more comfortable in cooperative, interdependent settings. Women's sexuality is exploited, their intelligence questioned, their roles limited and often confusing. They are bombarded with promises of a "better self" through the dieting, fashion, cosmetics and anti-aging industries. Most women feel unsupported by a culture with such shallow values! They want and deserve something more—something that gives their lives meaning in a deeper way.

It is this role within this society which is at different times limiting, confusing, frightening, and unfulfilling, that propels enormous numbers of women into the safety and numbness of food problems.

• Women are socialized in specific ways.

Generally speaking, in the course of growing up, women are taught to relate and behave in ways which are specific to our culture. This is called being "socialized" or "acculturated." Although strides have been made, many archaic ideas remain. Four of the most harmful lessons which can contribute to eating disorders are the following: (Buckroyd, 1996)

1. Women should mistrust their spontaneity and energy and instead be careful and cautious, especially about their own capabilities. Boys are allowed and encouraged to have far more physical freedom and to take more risks.

2. Women should not be too needy, and their needs come last. They should also anticipate the needs of

others, just as mothers anticipate the needs of babies and children.

3. Women should defer to others by letting others take the lead, therby giving up their opinions, and placing themselves in subordinate and auxiliary positions.

4. Women should be concerned with their appearance because they will be judged on it. At the same time, their bodies will be objectified and sexualized on a mass scale.

These lessons teach women that they have cultural "limitations." They become afraid to express themselves freely, and deny their own needs, strengths, opinions, and inherent beauty. Bulimia can be a distraction from feeling disconnected from one's own self.

• Adolescent women are particularly vulnerable.

The message that women should be concerned with their appearance is communicated to both sexes starting at birth, along the path through childhood, adolescence, and right into adulthood. Particularly when kids enter puberty, however, becoming more independent from their families and facing the culture at large, young girls are bombarded with images of female bodies as objects which are scrutinized unmercifully. They also become aware of stereotypical "feminine" traits, such as cleanliness, docility, unselfishness, politeness, and sometimes being a tease. By the time sexual game-playing starts, most of them already know that their bodies are tools for popularity and power, and that there is appropriate and inappropriate behavior associated with being a girl.

Also, a strange thing happens to girls at this age. Their sure sense of self, strong opinions, and unabashed involvement give way to powerlessness, insecurity, and doubts about their appearance. They are no longer cute little girls, they are budding sexual women. From a girl's perspective, this puts her in a vulnerable position with regard to men, and a competitive one with women. At a time when she is forging an identity, altering her body to fit everyone's expectations, including those of her culture, seems to be a reasonable way to please everyone. Many young women develop eating disorders when they fail their initial attempts at dieting and are faced with the fear that they will never be an "ideal" woman.

- **Having a female body in this society can be frightening.**

Men, for the most part, are more sexually driven than women, whether this trait is biologically inherited or learned from their environment. Women, on the other hand, are driven more by a deep desire to maintain connections with others. These two factors have created an environment of pervasive sexual abuse and harassment against women, both young and old, within our society which we are just beginning to face.

Recent statistics of sexual abuse and violence against women are staggeringly high. An eating disorder is a way of coping with the pain of that experience, "My body is my own. I am in control of what goes in and out of it." It can be an unconscious reenactment of the original abuse or a way to punish the body which was "to blame" for the assault. It can also be a way to distance one's self from one's body or numb the feelings associated with abuse or harassment. Ultimately, an eating disorder is a safe place to hide from the pain and fear of mistreatment.

• **Contemporary society denies the natural variety and function of women's bodies.**

"Becoming a woman" is for many an embarrassing, self-conscious affair, requiring daily self-scrutiny. Most feel required to shave their legs and underarms, hide their periods, and control body odors. Even women who have experienced the miracle of giving birth are driven to quickly flatten their stomachs afterwards, as though it had never happened! Denying women's deepest biological truth trivializes their lives. An eating disorder can ease the pain of being disconnected from this inner source of strength and meaning.

• **Women are expected to control their emotions.**

Many women with bulimia report fearing the intensity of bottled-up feelings. Consequently, many have little experience with their emotions or appetites for sex, food, or living. Some say that they cannot distinguish one feeling from another or that they swing back and forth from extreme highs to lows. Letting out their emotions would mean being engulfed by them or engulfing others. Females are expected to keep their anger in check—not even talk too much! Controlling their bodies, specifically food intake, becomes a concrete way to feel in control of this inner instability. Thinness becomes a measure of emotional control, and bulimia a way to insure it.

• **Women are frustrated in the work place.**

Although the women's movement has provided new opportunities for some fortunate women who have taken advantage, the majority of today's working women continue to be discriminated against in the male-dominated marketplace and political arena. Those who are able to land jobs in the areas of their interest and expertise are often paid less than men and are under tremendous pressure to perform. Also, as we said earlier, jobs which require a high degree of competition and supervision can be unsatisfying for many women who are more apt to thrive in an atmosphere of cooperation and mutuality.

In these cases, bulimia can be a symptom of a life devoid of meaning, creativity, or rewarding work. It can also help let off steam or provide a way to self-sabotage in order to avoid failure or intimacy in the workplace.

• **The media and money perpetuate the status quo.**

The extensive influence of the media is unquestionable. Images of women as sexual objects are endlessly reinforced via television, movies, magazines, newspapers, billboards, and consumer products, conveying to *both* sexes that women should be thin, pretty, and sexy. Billion dollar businesses depend on women feeling insecure about their appearance.

While a cover girl's photo or cosmetics advertisement does not cause a binge, these constant reminders that thinner equals better establishes values that lead to distorted ways of viewing food and the self. How can a woman feel good about who she is on the inside if everyone else seems to focus on the outside? Ironically, many of the thin actresses and models, who are paid enormous sums for their "look" and skinny bodies, are themselves struggling with eating disorders in an effort to remain marketable.

What special issues are faced by men with bulimia?

While the actual numbers of men with bulimia are unknown and are certainly less than for women, more men have bulimia than anyone thought in the early 80s, when information about this eating disorder first emerged. Current estimates are that at least 10% of individuals with eating disorders are males. However, much of the latest research on prevalence is based on small studies and lacks conclusive findings. Men can also develop anorexia nervosa; and unlike women, some become obsessed with getting larger and more muscular—a condition called "reverse anorexia" or "body dysmorphia" which can also become addictive.

Considering the issues that surround bulimia, such as guilt, shame, and low self-esteem, it is understandable that men might feel these emotions even more intensely when they have what has been generally regarded as a "women's" disease. For this reason, many bulimic men may have been reluctant to seek professional help. Those who use exercise addiction as a type of purge generally deny that they have a problem with food. Perfectionistic "low-fat eaters" hide their obsession behind a facade of health and fitness.

For the most part, men appear to become bulimic for the same kinds of reasons that women do. Some male athletes, such as wrestlers, jockeys and gymnasts, use bulimia to maintain or lose weight and become hooked on it, just as is the case for female athletes. Although contemporary thought suggests that more women are bulimic than men because society has traditionally placed more of an emphasis on women's appearance, men are increasingly encouraged to conform to a narrow range of body types. The gay community, in particular, is concerned with "lookism" and roughly 20% of male bulimics are gay (Andersen, 1999). Heavy male models are as rare as full-figured females, and men are encouraged to diet, undergo plastic surgery and alter their hair just like women.

Men are also under pressure to appear strong, in control, and independent, and as such, their roles in our culture have limitations and drawbacks, just like women's. Many have difficulty expressing feelings and have had little experience in emotionally intimate relationships. Most feel tremendous pressure to be in charge, to shoulder financial worries and be the foundation for their families and other responsibilities. Few would want to be labelled as obsessed with their appearance. All these situations might make them more susceptible to using bulimia as a coping mechanism, as well as extremely reluctant to seek help.

Most research concludes that there are far more similarities than differences when comparing men and women with bulimia. In addition to our pervasive, cultural diet-consciousness, other factors such as dysfunctional families, sexual abuse, low self-esteem, and lack of meaning in one's life contribute to the causes for becoming bulimic, regardless of gender. Recovery outcomes for each are also parallel.

Finding adequate therapy has its own unique concerns for men. Treatment options for women are plentiful and diverse, and only in recent years have programs been developed that are available solely for men. Therefore, finding professional support may require a lot of searching and may mean settling for a general men's or mixed bulimia support group.

Men might find it necessary to step outside the roles they've defined for themselves, and to interpret feminist recovery literature to meet their own needs. For instance, one aspect of feminism is valuing relationships between people rather than being separate from them. This might well apply to men who are encouraged to be so independent and competitive that they feel isolated from others and drawn to bulimia.

As a society, both men and women perpetuate negative stereotypes, and it is up to both sexes to learn how to relate to each other in fulfilling, nurturing ways. As you know, the language of this book primarily addresses women, but most of the underlying messages and suggested activities are also worthwhile for men.

How is bulimia related to sexual trauma?

Clinical studies are inconsistent in reporting the numbers of eating disorders patients that have been sexually abused, and there is some controversy about this. Figures for bulimics with a history of sexual abuse range from an astounding 7% to 70%, with a majority reporting that roughly 60% of bulimics have experienced some form of sexual abuse (Vanderlinden, 1996). Since all of these figures do not include individuals who have repressed the memories of their abuse, the actual incidence is undoubtedly higher than much of the research has shown.

It is important to be aware of the extremely sensitive nature of this topic, and that a self-help book such as this is not adequate "therapy" for healing these issues. With the understanding that victims need to work with a qualified therapist who has experience treating individuals suffering with both eating disorders and sexual trauma, I will present an overview on this subject. Also, although I am using the pronoun "she," incest and sexual abuse occur with startlingly high incidence among males, with similar consequences.

Being sexually assaulted, especially by a "trusted" adult, parent, or sibling, is a terrifying, confusing, horrific experience for anyone. It is an act of violence and betrayal so intense that just remembering it is agonizingly painful. In order to survive not only the trauma itself but also the memory of it, a victim might dissociate from the event and from those parts of herself which were present at that time. She may even consider the person being raped to be separate from herself, because the pain is too much for her to bear. Her emotional and physical survival depend on her not remembering the events or her feelings connected with what happened.

An eating disorder works to protect, repress, complete, divert, numb, or confuse these feelings and memories. Certainly it is not within a child's realm of possibility to blame the abuser for what happened, but even an adult will tend to blame herself for the attack, making her body the focus for hatred and control. Stuffing down food will stuff down the anger and silence the voice that cries out, "Don't do this to me!" Planning and executing a binge will numb anxieties and deny physical needs, such as hunger or affection. Being in charge of what does, and does not, go into the body is a way to symbolically regain that control which was lost during the original trauma.

The relationship with food makes it difficult to have full relationships with others, thus eliminating the risk of another betrayal. Depending on the individual's internal survival tools, being extremely large or thin, or even perceiving one's self as too large or too thin, is a way of keeping potential abusers at a distance. Finally, the painful and violent act of vomiting is a way of expressing and releasing rage and self-loathing.

Many victims of sexual abuse become promiscuous, masochistic, or even fantasize about rape during consenting lovemaking without realizing that they are hooked on the "high" of relief they experience by blocking out their assault. Likewise, they can repeat this "forbidden high" by bingeing and purging. Some bulimics compulsively follow rituals which might mirror repeated incidents, such as molestation from a babysitter every Saturday night or visits from a sibling when parents are out of the house. Forced eating and vomiting also parallel the act of forced oral sex. These repetitive behaviors may be an attempt on the part of the unconscious to complete the original abuse in the present. An even more upsetting eating pattern may be the result of Satanic rituals, which could involve swallowing excrement or blood. Given the appalling scope of sexual trauma within this context, it is apparent that an eating disorder can be a crucial mechanism for survival.

Although we are defining sexual abuse here in terms of more extreme behaviors, practically every woman has suffered sexual humiliation in some form or another. Their breasts have been "accidentally" brushed up against, their virginity has been the subject of male gossip, and they have been whistled or jeered at by strangers. In all of these cases, the female is victimized by the standard line, "She was asking for it." It is no coincidence that epidemic numbers of women also suffer from some type of food/weight conflict, the most common of which is dieting. Sadly, women's bodies have become their enemies instead of the natural wonder that they are.

Sexual trauma must be treated in a safe, trusted environment. Coming to terms with the experience, repressed or not, and returning the inner child to an experience of unconditional love and acceptance is a tremendous undertaking. It requires gentle understanding and patience by therapist and patient alike. Keep in mind that eliminating the binge-purge behavior without introducing healthy coping skills can result in a reliving of the original horror. Making some kind of peace with the nightmare that lies beneath the bulimic surface is best achieved with the guidance of a trained and skilled professional (Schwartz, 1996).

Working and uncovering the truth about my family, and the fact that I was incested, helped everything make sense. I saw how wounded I was, and how much pain and anger I worked dutifully to deny. I began to see that I had value, and that I was lovable and competent, but that I had not been treated that way by my parents. I realized that my eating disorder was motivated by my archaic need to protect my family, and that I was actually recreating my abuse.

When I was 12, my brother began sexually abusing me. I was overwhelmed with confusion and believed if I became fat, he might leave me alone. I think gaining 40 pounds in three months was also my way of saying, "Hey, there's something wrong here," without having to verbalize it.

My physical and sexual abuse began at an early age. Much of the abuse centered around food, with my father demanding favors for desserts. Some days, it was all right to leave food on my plate, others it wasn't. Food became my lasting enemy.

My Dad used to tell dirty jokes. At the time, we all laughed, but they were all demeaning to women. I wondered if he really thought about women, my mother, in that way, but I never asked him.

I had a swallowing problem due to being forced into oral sex. I would spit out all of my food, even liquids. I had been through every medical test in the book because the doctors thought there was something wrong with my throat. After four years of therapy, that problem is finally gone; but, it comes back at times of high stress or when memories surface.

It's important for parents, therapists, doctors, and the public to know that women who were sexually abused are in a lot of pain. Their eating disorder is a way of dealing with all of the feelings—rage, anger, secrecy, fear, betrayal, powerlessness and many others. An eating disorder is a feeling disorder because it helps you handle your feelings.

How does bulimia affect my relationships?

Bulimia is sometimes referred to as a relationship disorder because it does, to a large degree, disrupt normal, healthy relationships. Individuals with bulimia gradually withdraw from others until their obsession with food becomes practically the sole one. Also, most of our beliefs about ourselves, like whether or not we are good people or if we have to be thin to be loved, are born in our most important relationships. The eating disorder primarily serves as a protective device which insures that past hurts on these intimate issues are not remembered or repeated in the present.

As children, the ways in which we are treated by our parents, other adults, our peers and our community-at-large tell us something about us. These relationships are the foundation for our feelings of significance, competence, and ability to be loved. Un-

fortunately, many of us have been abused emotionally and physically by the very people entrusted with our lives. With our child's
mind, we cannot believe that the fault lies with our caretakers, so
we blame ourselves. We even have a hard time believing that our
culture, the largest family of all, might not be such a good one.

This is not to imply that eating disorders develop only in
households where there is violence or physical abuse. Being repeatedly ignored or undervalued can be as damaging to a child's
self-image as being incested. Children who do not feel loved or
safe in any type of family don't trust their own actions. They will
then look outside themselves for cues on how to behave. As a
result, their relationships will be "other-directed" and founded in
low self-esteem.

Bulimia, which often begins as an innocent attempt to gain
thinness and thus please others, is an example of this other-directed behavior. The person with bulimia is not following her
own heart, she is reacting to what is going on around her. While
it appears to be protecting her by preserving a false front and a
sense of safety, it also keeps people at a distance. Bulimics interact with people knowing that they can withdraw at any time to
their familiar, repetitive behaviors. Even when a bulimic appears
to be present in conversation, her mind can be light years away,
in the last or next binge.

Certain aspects of bulimia are particularly detrimental to forming honest, fulfilling relationships. Obviously, maintaining a happy,
competent facade on the outside, while feeling anxious or depressed on the inside, is an effort and a distraction. The binge
and purge behaviors are done secretly, usually shrouded by feelings of guilt and shame. Mood swings and lying are common
characteristics. Stealing, which was mentioned by 37% of the people
who answered our survey, reinforces low self-esteem and hiding.

Focusing on thinness encourages competition between women instead of support, and emphasizes the sexual nature of relationships with men instead of affection or respect.

Over time, a bulimic's relationship with food will come to supersede all other relationships. As one person who responded to our survey said, "Bulimia is a friend who does not criticize, judge, compete, or reject." However, bulimic behavior cannot love us the way we need to be loved. It does not nurture, support, or fulfill us and the deepest inner level, as anyone who has gorged and purged themselves over and over will testify. It is a tenuous short-term solution for buried long-term pain, creating loneliness and isolation in its wake.

Giving up bulimic behavior is extremely frightening for someone who has little experience being close to others. It means risking rejection and facing feelings of worthlessness, but the payoffs are obvious—honesty, trust, fun, intimacy, and love. As the section in this book on getting support emphasizes, an open, trusting relationship with even one person can be a crucial factor in recovery. Many people found this trust in therapy; others found it with parents, lovers, spouses, and friends.

The very nature of an eating disorder prevents the development of relationships. How could I have a relationship with someone based on honesty and truth if I was constantly lying about how much I ate, didn't eat, exercised, or purged?

When I am in love or working on intimacy, my eating habits normalize, but when I have no close relationships or involvement with others, I feel like I am starving. Food reduces the anxiety, and masks the feelings. Only working on intimacy stops this pattern. For me, relationship-building is essential to recovery.

Basically, my life became a massive cover-up. Any lie or deception that protected my freedom to binge-purge was okay, and I'd always placed a high value on honesty prior to this! My relationships with my family members deteriorated as they caught me in numerous lies. They couldn't trust most of what I said. I actually believed that the reason my sisters were tracking me around the house, in an attempt to stop my vomiting, was because they were jealous that I was finally thinner than they were!

When I went out with friends, I was so detached from what was going on that all I could do was calculate how fast I needed to get to the bathroom to vomit. I had no real interest in the people around me; but, through therapy, that's all changing now.

I recall on many occasions, turning on my answering machine, settling down to plates of my favorite binge foods, and listening to friends leave messages, while I frantically shoveled in food. Food had become more important than my friends. Food was my BEST friend.

As I became more comfortable with myself, I saw my life change in many ways. I found myself surrounded by friends who really liked me. And they were happy people, not miserable and depressed like my old friends.

I have learned how to say "no" to people, and earned a lot of respect for doing so. I was always afraid of what would happen if I disagreed or wanted something to be different. Now I feel worth having an opinion.

Is it the same as anorexia nervosa?

For many years bulimia was considered to be one type of anorexic behavior. Certainly, in both cases, the relationship with food is a symptom of other serious problems and many other similarities do exist. By recognizing bulimia as a separate disorder in 1980, however, the American Psychiatric Association identified a much larger group than those who could be clinically classified as strictly anorexic.

The fourth edition of the American Psychiatric Association's Diagnostic and Statistical Manual of Mental Disorders (APA, 1994) lists four criteria that an individual must meet in order to be diagnosed as anorexic, generalized as follows:

A. The individual maintains a body weight that is about 15% below normal for age, height, and body type.

B. The individual has an intense fear of gaining weight or becoming fat, even though they are underweight. Paradoxically, losing weight can make this fear of gaining even worse.

C. The individual has a distorted body image. Some may feel fat all over, others recognize that they are generally thin but see specific body parts (particularly the stomach and thighs) as being too fat. Their self-worth is based on their body size and shape. They deny that their low body weight is serious cause for concern.

D. In women, there is an absence of at least three consecutive menstrual cycles. A woman also meets this criteria if her period occurs only while she is taking a hormone pill (including, but not limited to, oral contraceptives).

The DSM-IV also differentiates between two specific types of anorexia nervosa. "Restricting Type" denotes individuals who lose weight primarily by reducing their overall food intake through dieting, fasting and/or exercising excessively. "Binge-Eating/Purging Type" describes those who regularly binge (consume large amounts of food in short periods of time), and purge through self-induced vomiting, excessive exercise, fasting, the abuse of diuretics, laxatives, and enemas, or any combination of these measures (Hall and Ostroff, 1998).

Although some anorexics also purge after eating, anorexia nervosa is generally characterized by self-starvation. In general, anorexics reject food, have lower body weight, often begin younger, and are socially and sexually less mature. In contrast, the majority of bulimics' weight appears closer to normal, most began purging in their late teens or early twenties (many anorexics turn to bulimia), and are more socially outgoing. Also, as noted, the DSM-IV criteria includes amenorrhea, which is generally rare amongst bulimics, who nevertheless, frequently report irregular menses.

Hospitalization is often necessary for anorexics, who have a higher fatality rate: 5-20% of anorexics die from complications related to the disease (Zerbe, 1995). There is no definitive data for bulimia fatality statistics, but the clinical impression is that they are low, and not as high as for anorexia nervosa.

There are, as mentioned above, similarities in the issues underlying anorexia nervosa and bulimia. Individuals with the disorders share an overconcern with the size of their bodies and what they have or have not eaten. They are focused on an inner empty place, which can be viewed in physical, emotional, social or spiritual terms. Both use the control of food to handle intense feelings of different kinds, such as depression, anger, rejection, loneliness, selfishness, fear of independence or dependence, and love. Each also uses food to avoid situations where there is a potential for conflict, disapproval, or failure. Ultimately, both use food to express something that they feel is unacceptable or they are unable to express directly.

However, while a binge and purge can give a bulimic the courage to face the world, not-eating is empowering to an anorexic. Although some anorexics engage in purges if they eat more than they consider safe, not-eating remains their primary tool for self-preservation. Recovery for these individuals is less a matter of avoiding a binge than it is eating enough to be healthy. But the bottom line for both remains to be able and willing to care for themselves with appropriate amounts of food (not starving or stuffing) in a healthy, self-nurturing way.

What is a typical binge?

"Typical" depends entirely on the individual. The size and frequency can vary as well as the type of purge and the length of time between sessions. A binge is really whatever causes a person to feel guilty. Typical binges, however, share two characteristics—the consumption of an excessive amount of food and feelings of being out of control.

Many bulimics have said that they can "relate to" my binges, one of which I've described in the Introduction. Frequently I started a binge while in the course of eating what I thought to be a "good" or "safe" meal. For example, I may have gone to a salad bar and carefully allowed myself a moderate portion. As I ate the salad, I would begin to feel guilty about the calories in the salad dressing or the fact that I had taken croutons. At one point in the meal, I would decide I had eaten one bite too many. Rather than stop eating, I'd think, "What's the difference. I've already gone too far. I'll do a binge, and none of the calories will matter after I vomit." It never occurred to me that there were "issues" driving this bizarre behavior.

If I had my choice, I would eat sweets and refined carbohydrates. A single binge might include: a quart of ice cream, a bag of cookies, a couple of batches of brownies, a dozen donuts, and a few candy bars. When I was desperate, though, I would binge on anything: oatmeal, cottage cheese, carrots, or day-old rolls that I fished out of the trash from what was to be my last-ever binge.

My stomach stretched so much that I looked pregnant, and I usually postponed vomiting for about 30 minutes of numbness. Then I'd stick my fingers down my throat until I had vomited everything that would come up. The whole episode lasted about an hour, and I often felt very weak and dizzy afterwards. I did not abuse laxatives, enemas, or diuretics, although some others with bulimia do.

What are the medical dangers?

Although bulimia rarely results in death, it can occur. Excessive vomiting leads to electrolyte imbalance. Electrolytes, which are chemicals in the body like potassium, chloride and sodium, help regulate heart beat. When they are depleted by purging or dehydration, heart arrhythmia—irregular heart beat—often takes place. Sometimes this is not serious and subsides when proper health and nutrition is restored, but for others it can lead to death from cardiac arrest. Kidney failure is another possible life-threatening side-effect of low potassium. Vomiting can be fatal due to choking or if the esophagus or bronchial passage is ruptured.

The most common medical problems for bulimics include rotten teeth, constipation, bloating and other digestive disorders, infected or swollen glands known as "chipmunk cheeks," blisters in the throat, icy hands and feet, and fluid depletion. Other potentially serious, though generally rare, complications are abnormalities in the endocrine and gastrointestinal systems, anemia, internal bleeding, hypoglycemia, irregular menstrual periods or amenorrhea, osteoporosis, myopathy, and irregularities in brain imaging.

Some bulimics use syrup of ipecac, detergents, or foreign objects to induce vomiting—all of which are extremely dangerous. Ipecac, a horrible tasting liquid, is used to treat poison victims, and its abuse can produce muscle weakness or cardiac arrest (Mitchell, 1997; Mickley, 1999).

Laxative abuse can irritate intestinal nerve endings, which can inhibit them from triggering contractions. Heavy use of laxatives or enemas removes protective mucus from the intestinal lining, which can result in bowel infections. The lower bowel can lose muscle tone, becoming limp and unable to produce contractions. Dehydration and fluid imbalances can occur with the same side-effects as listed above. Also, laxative abusers can have rectal pain, gas, constipation or diarrhea (or both), and bowel tumors.

Although not directly linked, individuals with eating disorders may tend to have other medical illnesses, including diabetes mellitus, cystic fibrosis, inflammatory bowel diseases such as Crohn's disease, and thyroid disease. Diabetics with bulimia often misuse their insulin, which can be life-threatening (Bock, 1999; Zerbe, 1995).

It is difficult, if not impossible, to know which bulimics are at greatest risk for developing any of these specific conditions. Certainly, the longer someone has bulimia, the more likely they are to experience associated medical problems. However, even someone who has only started to purge faces the possibility of serious physical consequences, even death.

Many bulimics have concerns about getting or being pregnant. Some fear that their vomiting will harm the child or that they will get too fat. Although information on pregnancy and eating disorders is limited, what we do know is:

1. Although women with disordered eating are more likely to deliver babies that are small, major birth defects do not accompany bulimia or anorexia nervosa.

2. Since a mother who purges has a separate digestive system than her fetus, the child is generally not harmed. However, poor nutrition and negative frame of mind are unhealthy for mother and child.

3. For women in treatment, some antidepressants can be used but others should be avoided. In any case, they should check with their doctors about the specific medications that they are taking.

4. A large percentage of women experience remission of their bulimic symptoms while they are pregnant. They may feel that their bodies belong to their babies during pregnancy, and thus eliminate unhealthy behaviors. However during the postpartum period they are likely to return to their bulimia, especially faced with their added weight.

5. The birth of a child also brings up other emotional issues for bulimic women, which include mother/child relationships, how the eating disorder will affect parenting, sexuality and attractiveness, separation conflicts, and worries over proper feeding for baby. These should all be addressed for the welfare of the mother and child (Yager, 1997; Zerbe, 1995).

What thoughts and feelings are associated with it?

Eating disorders are *feeling* disorders. The rigid rules and rituals of bulimic behavior are a definite way to distance one's self from feelings that seem unmanageable, overwhelming, or just plain terrifying. These can be as nightmarish as the fear that comes from memories of abuse, the quiet pain of being unloved or considered unimportant, or feelings that are buried in past events or fresh from one's daily life. A binge pushes away all feelings by providing something else on which to focus.

Eventually, bulimics use no other way of handling their feelings *except* to binge and purge. This is what they describe when they say they feel powerless. What's more, the illness brings with it a whole new set of complications that mask the old feelings and often make them worse. For example, a person who is afraid of others may use bulimia to keep her distance by hiding her embarrassing thoughts and rituals. Or someone who feels incompetent may perfect the art of throwing up, while attempting little else. In this way, whatever precipitated the binge-purge behavior is effectively denied, and in the long run, buried beneath fresh shame and guilt.

Most initial lessons about feelings are acquired at an early age and have a profound impact. Some families do not express or know how to handle a free range of emotions, especially "negative" ones, such as anger, disappointment or even disagreement. Others have strict rules for controlling which emotions can be expressed and what modes of expression are permitted. Children in these types of families learn that they should monitor and protect their feelings, and in many cases deny them altogether. With no experience identifying and talking about them, a bulimic may not even know exactly *what* she is feeling, or might assume that her feelings are bad and she is bad for having them. She might fear other people's feelings, as well, and work hard to insure that they are not upset in any way.

Eventually these unvoiced feelings will find expression in other ways, such as through an eating disorder. In fact, many bulimics misinterpret a wide range of emotions as hunger. Most say that they feel depressed, disconnected and powerless most of the time. The cyclical nature of the bulimic binges also applies to feelings which, in the space of a few hours, can move from *worthlessness* (low self-esteem), to *powerlessness* (I have no control over my life), *effectiveness* (I can get rid of these feelings), a *"high"* from the release of the purge, *hope* (that this binge might be the last), and finally the return to feelings of *worthlessness*.

Bulimia is also a *thinking* disorder in that sufferers are trapped in harmful thought patterns. One example is "black and white thinking," where everything is divided into extreme categories. For example, foods are either "good" or "bad," bodies are either "fat" or "thin," and not being in-control means being completely out-of-control. Other patterns are magnifying problems, magical and dramatic thinking, constantly comparing one's self to others, and taking remarks or situations too personally. Some bulimics also seem to hold a generally negative attitude towards life, which influences all aspects of their experience. Most think that they are worthless, as evidenced by the size of their bodies.

Individuals with bulimia typically harbor a set of deeply-held core ideas upon which other harmful conclusions are drawn. For instance, the belief that being fat is bad will also mean that food is bad, that having a large body is a sign of failure, and that self-indulgence is a sign of weakness. Believing that "I am a bad person," to which many bulimics adhere, makes possible the thoughts "There is no reason to take care of myself," and "No one can love me." This sets up an entire system of values and ideas upon which they are constantly monitoring and judging themselves, and sometimes others. Their minds do what is referred to as "spinning," or going over and over the same negative thoughts. These endless, automatic "tapes" in the mind make it impossible for bulimics to hear anything else, much less their own inner wisdom.

All these negative feelings and thoughts must be brought to light and challenged in recovery. This can be at once a frightening, rejuvenating, exhausting, rewarding experience, which is why it is best done with the guidance of a therapist.

I can easily see how, during stressful times of your life, you seek some kind of comfort. I found this in food. Others find it in drugs and alcohol.

Before I started therapy, I never associated my desire to binge with my emotions. I always felt it was an uncontrollable desire for huge amounts of food. Now I understand the binge takes the place of allowing myself to feel any emotions.

When I feel sad, troubled, panic, anger or loneliness, this disease jumps out on me like a Jack-in-the-box. I find it scary because I also feel helpless and not in control. Then again, the mental "numbness" blocks out all the emotions and makes me forget about all my problems. It's not worth it, though.

What other behaviors do bulimics share?

People with eating disorders have compulsive personalities; the rituals they create are safe and familiar places to reside. Many of the rituals revolve around food and body image, such as arranging food on their plates, excessive exercise, eating systematically, looking in the mirror, and obsessive calorie counting. Some behaviors are not related to food, such as always knowing where the nearest bathroom is, avoiding people, lying, keeping secrets, kleptomania, and compulsive shopping.

Most bulimics take exhaustive steps to cover up their symptoms. During the five years of my first marriage, my husband never found out about my closely-guarded secrets. No one knew! Covering my tracks was part of my daily routine. Lying about food was second nature to me. For example, if I went to the same grocery two days in a row to buy large quantities of binge food, I would tell the checker that I was a nursery school teacher buying snacks for the children. My rituals included a preoccupation with scales, mirrors, and trying on clothes. I used to weigh myself before and after binges to be sure that I gained no weight. (At one point in my recovery, I took a hammer to the scale!) I could not pass a mirror without judging every slight bulge or hair out of place.

In our survey, 37% of the bulimics mentioned kleptomania as a symptom. Obviously, stealing is one way to offset the cost of food, but there is more to kleptomania than just basic economics. Both compulsive shopping and stealing are ways to "fill up" without eating, as well as to symbolically fulfill unmet emotional needs. Also, stealing from other people can be a way to communicate negative feelings without using words.

In my case, I felt unworthy and incapable of affording "nice" things, although I spent vast amounts on food. I wanted love and attention, and not knowing how to get those emotional rewards, I settled for the temporary satisfaction of new things. Sometimes I just wanted the rush of doing something I shouldn't. The women in our survey had similar experiences. Their stealing ranged from candy bars to larger, more expensive items. Most of those who stole also indicated that it was not too difficult a pattern to change. A few women were arrested, then stopped immediately, such as this one:

I stopped stealing after I got caught with a chicken in my purse!

What does it feel like to binge-vomit?

In answering this question, it is important to remember that bulimia serves a purpose for the person using it. In other words, they would not be binge eating and purging if it made them feel worse rather than better. Particularly in the early stages, when purging is excused as a way to lose weight or maintain low weight, bulimia provides a false sense of self-esteem, competence, and control. In the later stages, giving it up means understanding the difference between what is real and true and what is not. It also means choosing what is real.

The mental "numbness" and physical "high" are important reasons that the binge-vomiting behavior itself becomes so addictive. In fact, many women from our survey who were compulsive about food were also alcoholics, or came from families where substance abuse existed. There have been several studies on the comorbidity of eating disorders and other addictions, and they have shown that between 9% and 55% of bulimics are also alcoholic or abuse drugs. They also become addicted to diet pills, diuretics, and laxatives (Mitchell, 1997).

Friends and loved-ones should know that vomiting from a binge is not the same thing as vomiting when you are sick. The person with bulimia doesn't feel sick, she feels desperate, driven. Bingeing and purging temporarily removes stress, like a drug. All focus is on the cycle, from trying to avoid a binge, giving in to the urge, planning, and execution. After a vomiting purge, there is also a physical "high" from the pressure of being upside down and exhausting physical effort. Feelings of cleanliness, renewal, relaxation, mindlessness, and emotional numbness are common. There may be sexual feelings from the emerging, private excitement, complete involvement, fullness, stroking, and sudden release.

In my case, in the calm after the purging storm, I promised myself that I would never binge again, adding feelings of hope and renewal to the cycle. But shortly thereafter, I always started anew. For more than five years, I binged and vomited four or five times—and more—practically every day. Several surveyed women commented about the drug-like aspect of bulimia:

I like the high and then the numbness. Once I begin a binge, there is no stopping me.

When I first tried to give up my bulimic behaviors, I began to drink more alcohol. I was substituting one escape for another. I would get so depressed over my drinking that I would finally binge. I joined Alcoholics Anonymous, have been sober five months, and find my bulimia much more manageable. Until I quit drinking I kept having recurrent episodes of my old bulimic behavior.

No matter how down and depressed you feel, think of food as a temporary filling or "high." Find something permanent, because after you purge, you'll feel the same or even worse. Why waste your time?

How do I know if I have bulimia?

Have we been talking about you? I binged and vomited daily for nine years without thinking I had a problem, although that was before bulimia had been given a name. I came across the very first magazine article about "bulimarexia" and was shocked to discover that there were other people who had the same eating behavior as mine.

Whether you binge and purge daily or only occasionally, or if you overeat and then exercise compulsively or engage in strict dieting, you are still abusing your body in a bulimic manner. Actually, even if you are only obsessive in your thoughts about weight, diet, and food, you still have a problem with food, even if you do not meet the clinical definition for anorexia or bulimia.

To address the problems of individuals who do not fit the strict criteria, the American Psychiatric Association established a new category in the DSM-IV, "Eating Disorders Not Otherwise Specified" (EDNOS). Some of the symptoms of EDNOS include binge eating without purging, meeting all of the criteria for anorexia except the individual has regular menses or is close to normal weight, having bulimic symptoms with less frequency than twice a week or for a duration of less than three months, purging after eating relatively small portions, or chewing and spitting out the food rather than swallowing.

Just about everyone enjoys an occasional large meal (holiday

binges!), but an obsession is an escape. If you have constant negative thoughts about food and your body, you have a problem
regardless of its clinical classification, and I urge you to face it.

How long does it take to get better?

That's up to you. The behavior does not suddenly stop without an effort. In fact, it is addictive enough to continue as a lifelong obsession. I have corresponded with a woman in her sixties
who has been bulimic for more than forty years! In the past, so
little was known about bulimia that people commonly continued
for years before seeking help. Now, there are national and local
organizations, treatment facilities, private therapists, support groups,
and books solely devoted to eating disorders.

There are a few necessary steps to recovery. The first is acknowledging that you have a problem and making the decision
to change. For some people, prolonged therapy, or even hospitalization, is necessary. Generally, overcoming bulimia takes time
and a firm commitment, and increased time, effort and determination will make it happen faster.

The time it takes to stop the bingeing behavior varies with
each individual. I have heard of people who have gone "cold
turkey," stopping instantly, and of others who have decreased the
number of binges slowly over a period of months or years while
they worked on the underlying issues. Stopping the binge-purge
behavior is like opening Pandora's box. Within are the reasons
why the bulimia began and took hold, as well as those it has
created anew. These all need to be resolved.

I am often asked how long it took me to recover. I spent a
year and a half working to stop the actual binge-purge behavior.

There was a time when only one binge each day seemed like an impossible goal, but days extended into weeks, and eventually my goal was to not binge for a month at a time. Ridding myself of the obsessive thoughts about food and my body took longer because I had to confront the issues that led me to become bulimic in the first place.

Stopping the behavior was only one aspect of recovery, though. I had goals related to my emotional life as well, such as improving my relationship with my parents, making more friends, being able to handle conflicts, and knowing what I needed and being able to articulate that to the people closest to me. I also had goals related to my body image, because I wanted to be able to love the body that I was born with no matter what its size or shape, and I wanted to stop being judgemental about other people's bodies. It was three or four years before I considered myself able to do that. A few years after that, I had stopped all bulimic behavior and had moved from being a basically negative person to a basically happy one. I didn't expect to ever go back to the way it was again, and called myself completely "cured."

So, there were many aspects to my recovery. Now, when someone asks me how long it took me to get better, I say that I am always working on my "betterment," primarily my spiritual life at this point. However, I have had no bulimic symptoms, thoughts or feelings whatsoever for many years. These days, I find it difficult to even remember my struggle with bulimia. I have not binged for about twenty years, and I do not think about returning to it. There are times, especially during menstruation, when I crave and eat more food than usual, especially chocolate. This is nothing like the eating binges when I was bulimic, either in content or quality.

Also, I was recently diagnosed with hyperthyroidism. At first, I didn't know why my body was speeded up or why I lost some weight and was hungry all the time. I just went with it, often consuming five meals a day until my condition was finally discovered. After treatment, I am gaining the weight back, and I feel ecstatic to be back in what feels like my "old, familiar" body. I can tell when I am at a healthy weight (not a particular weight!) and it feels good.

Not everyone agrees that you can be "cured" of an eating disorder. Some experts believe that bulimia is an addiction and that abstinence is the only way to prevent future relapse. They stress the addictive nature of certain types of foods which trigger responses that lead to bingeing. Like alcoholism, a complete cure is not possible because you will always be prone to bulimia, even if you do not practice the binge-purge behavior again. They would say that you are always "in recovery."

I know that this abstinence approach does work for many people, but I personally wanted to *lessen* food's power over me. I wanted to be completely free to eat anything I wanted. And so, my recovery focused on what is called the "legalized" approach to food. Instead of restricting, advocates of this approach stress differentiating stomach hunger from emotional hunger and fulfilling both accordingly. They emphasize getting satisfaction from eating what your body wants and suggest that when a preoccupation with eating and weight ends, bingeing stops as well.

In spite of my personal experience, I recommend many therapists and facilities who promote the abstinence approach, as well as those which do not. The information in this book applies to bulimics interested in recovery regardless of their stance on this issue. I do not advocate any specific modality of treatment—whatever works for you, do it!

It may be necessary to depend on another behavior, such as regularly-scheduled phone conversations with friends, or going to support group meetings to relieve tension or distract yourself. There is always the possibility that you will just trade one compulsivity for another. However, if you continually ask yourself if the steps you are taking are in a more positive direction, gradually you will be able to let go of all compulsivity. There will come a time when days pass without any fears associated with what you eat or look like. Remember, you are a worthwhile and important soul whose bulimia has served you in many ways. Be patient and gentle, work hard, and let it go.

Can medication help in recovery?

Even the strongest proponents of drug therapy do not recommend treatment based entirely on medication. No "magic pill" can fully resolve the emotional and spiritual issues underlying their bulimic behavior. Still, recent scientific data does support the use of antidepressants for the treatment of select patients with bulimia as part of a complete program administered by a treatment team. A consistent finding of many studies is that cognitive-behavioral psychotherapy alone is superior to solely using antidepressants, and sometimes the combination of medication and psychotherapy is even more effective (Garfinkel, 1997).

This is a controversial subject among clinicians. Most agree that individuals with eating disorders have mood disturbances, and many argue that bulimia is related to major affective disorder, the psychiatric family under which major depression is classified. Evidence also suggests that the cause of eating disorders might be traced to hereditary, genetic, and biological factors, including abnormalities of the hypothalamus, a gland in the brain which regulates many bodily functions.

Fluoxetine (brand name Prozac®) is the most widely-used antidepressant for bulimia, and many patients and therapists report good results from it as well as others, such as tricyclics (TCA's) and monoamine oxidase inhibitors (MAO's). However, antidepressants do not work for everyone, nor will any kind of treatment. Mood stabilizers, such as lithium carbonate, anxiolytics, and opiate antagonists have generally not been found to be effective in the treatment of bulimia (Garfinkel, 1997).

Some bulimics have responded well to drug treatment and have reduced the cravings to binge within weeks. Many of these patients have a history of depression, although being caught in the cycle of bulimic behavior can certainly cause depression as well. Some bulimics benefit from these medications because of chemical changes in their bodies related to hunger and satiety. Draw your own conclusions by consulting with a professional trained in the pharmacological treatment of bulimia.

Many people in our survey had experience with drug therapy. Close to 60% of those who had used antidepressants found them helpful in recovery. Several women indicated that drug therapy decreased their cravings to binge, allowing the issues that fueled the binge-purge behavior to surface.

Two of many psychiatrists I tried were biochemically oriented, and willing to modify pharmaceutical rules based on their own experience. We kept trying different doses and medicines until something worked.

I started using Prozac, and it really helped me. My urge to binge lessened practically overnight. It made me feel more ready for therapy.

I am being treated with Parnate (an MAO inhibitor) which has changed my life. It offers a "normal" mood, as well as freedom from binges. Of course, therapy in conjunction with medication is the ideal situation, and I'm trying that too. I don't think one without the other would do.

How do I learn to eat correctly?

Just as there is no one road to recovery, there is no one way to eat correctly. Every individual body is different, and deciding what and how much to eat will ultimately be up to you. In the early stages of recovery, however, when emotions are high and thoughts are spinning, food decisions are extremely difficult, sometimes immobilizing. It is helpful to have some plan with which you feel comfortable as you embark on new eating patterns. A qualified dietician or nutritionist, working in conjunction with your therapist, can help you with this. (See Chapter Six, "Healthy Eating and Healthy Weight.")

As I indicated earlier, there are two main approaches to the food behaviors in recovery from bulimia. People who use the abstinence approach eliminate certain foods from their diet and stick to a food plan. This enables them to avoid those foods which might trigger fears about weight gain or binges, such as sweets, processed, or fried foods. One common practice is to have three, well-planned meals each day and up to three healthy snacks.

The other orientation encourages people to eat whatever food they want, in moderate portions, when they are physically hungry. This is a more spontaneous approach and for this reason can be extremely difficult for someone new to recovery, requiring a new awareness of hunger cues and permission to eat that which was previously considered "bad," without guilt or loss of control. Most therapists recommend a more externally-structured eating plan at first, and a slow introduction to a more internally-guided plan.

It is hard even for a normal eater to make choices these days. The four food groups appear to be fast, frozen, fat, and fried—poor choices for anyone! Many restaurants serve overly large portions of fatty, sugary, processed food. With rare exceptions, fruits and vegetables are chemically treated, poultry and livestock are pumped with growth hormones, and much of our seafood swims in polluted waters. Finally, millions of dollars are spent promoting diet plans with powdery meal-substitutes or brand-name processed foods. What is considered healthy one week has warnings the next. Recovering bulimics have a particularly difficult time wading through this muck in order to learn how to eat nutritious meals.

Eating correctly obviously means not binge-eating or feeling badly about what you have eaten. It does mean following a relatively healthy, nutritious diet, allowing one's self the freedom to eat occasional treats without guilt or fear.

A healthy, well-balanced diet includes complex carbohydrates, protein, fat, vitamins, and minerals. Carbohydrates are the body's primary energy source and are crucial to the functioning of the red blood cells, brain, and central nervous system. Therefore, whole grains are an excellent source, as is pasta, rice, and starchy vegetables, such as potatoes. Protein also provides energy, and if enough carbohydrates are eaten, protein is used to build and repair tissue and help maintain adequate immune system function. Animal products provide "complete" proteins, but grains and legumes (such as rice and beans) can be adequately combined within a 24 hour period to form "complementary" proteins, which are essential for vegetarian diets. The body also needs fat to provide and absorb fat-soluble vitamins, fatty acids, and to slow the emptying of food from the stomach, which gives a feeling of fullness. Good sources are seeds (such as sunflower seeds) and unsaturated oils. A balanced diet, with plenty of variety, will provide the vitamins and minerals needed, although supplements may be appropriate. For more information, consult a professional or books on nutrition (not diet books).

Often, individuals with eating problems are well aware of these basic nutritional facts, but have difficulty acting upon them. This is because food represents much more than fuel and the act of eating symbolic of deeper issues. Changing your eating behavior may require trial and error over time in order to find what changes you are ready to make at the different stages of your progress.

Eating normally means enjoying what I eat. It also means loving myself enough to nourish my body with healthy, adequate nutrition.

To normal eaters, food is just food; it's not a substitute for something missing in your life, or a way to stuff feelings.

There are no more "good" or "bad" foods. I eat when I'm physically hungry, and stop when I'm comfortably satisfied. I can eat the foods I enjoy whenever I am hungry for them, and I am more aware of the taste and texture. I no longer binge as a result of deprivation.

I no longer binge or purge, but I also have to watch how much I eat, and I abstain from certain foods such as wheat, flour, hard cheese, and crispy, salty things like potato chips or rice cakes.

Eating normally is being able to eat anything I want, in moderation, with anyone I want. Now, I enjoy going out to eat with my husband and friends.

If I quit purging, will I gain weight?

There is no single answer to this question that is true for everyone. Some people gain weight when they stop purging, others lose or stay the same. This question is of obvious concern for most people with bulimia, but it brings up another, more relevant question: Why do you care? Whether you gain or lose weight is not as important as whether you can become self-accepting regardless of your weight or shape. (See Chapter Six, "Healthy Eating and Healthy Weight.")

Currently, the harmful message that thinness has innate value permeates every level of our society, although this has not always been the case. While there have been societal standards of beauty within every culture and time, emphasis has been increasingly placed on thinness in Westernized countries since the late '60s, particularly for women. Contemporary actresses and models, who represent the "ideal" woman are the thinnest 5-10% of the general public. Consequently, 90-95% of women are pressured to lose weight (Seid, 1994). So ingrained is the value of thinness that dieting has become an accepted part of their lives. One study showed that 42% of girls in the 1st through 3rd grades want to be thinner (Collins, 1991). Another showed that 51% of nine and ten year-old girls feel better about themselves when they are dieting; 9% of nine years olds have vomited to lose weight; 81% of ten year olds are afraid of being fat (Mellin, 1992).

A thin body has become a panacea, with both implied and actual rewards. We asked people who have had food problems to list their gut reactions to the words "thin" and "fat." "Thin" was associated with goodness, power, success, glamor, comfort, control, happiness, approval, attraction, friendship, love, and perfection. "Fat" indicated the opposite: panic, anger, self-hate, inferiority, unworthiness, unhappiness, loneliness, frustration, disgust, desperation, laziness, rejection, lack of control, ugliness, sloppiness, and failure! As a culture, we have been brainwashed. So much so that we can no longer separate the uniqueness of a person from the meanings connoted by the size of their bodies. This creates prejudice, the ultimate result of which is discrimination against people with large bodies. Naturally, you are worried about gaining weight!

The fact is that bodies come in all shapes and sizes and every person has a genetically programmed "natural" weight which is most healthy for them. This is called "set point." It is the weight at which they feel best, are neither eating too much or too little, and have a balanced metabolism. This ideal weight is a lot different than the one that is found on a standardized table. It is unique to every person. Actually, one's set point is a range of between about five to ten pounds. (See Chapter Seven, "Healthy Eating and

Healthy Weight.") Even a large body can be fit when it is at its set point—getting healthy food and regular, moderate exercise.

You can find your body on your family tree and there is not much you can do about it! Research has consistently shown that fat people, on the average, do not eat more than those who are thin. Biologically thin, adopted children in households with large adoptive parents do not grow up fat, or visa versa. Genetically thin people who are overfed do not become fat (Ellis-Ordway, 1999). In adoptive families, there is no relationship between the weights of the parents and children. Studies of twins also demonstrates that heredity accounts for about 70% of fatness (Foreyt, 1992).

In answer to the original question, frightening though it may be, many bulimics who resume normal eating do gain some weight while their metabolism adjusts to normal and they replenish their cellular water supply. *Eventually, they will level off at the weight that is genetically correct for their particular body.* At the same time, they are making the commitment to gain happiness, peace of mind, feelings of wholeness and integrity, as well as take care of themselves emotionally and physically. Interestingly, many individuals from our survey discovered that when they gave up dieting and the need to be thin, their bodies came to rest at weights that were acceptable, comfortable, beautiful, and unique. They were not necessarily thin.

I used to weigh myself at least 25 times a day. Now, I have not been on a scale for over two years. Eating disordered people like myself are so hung up on numbers. What should count is how you feel, not a number on the scale. It's hard to break the scale habit, but my advice to anyone is, don't weigh yourself at all!

I'm content with myself and realize I don't have to be skinny any longer. My health is more important to me than the image of "model thin."

Nothing could hurt me as much as being called "fat." It's only now, with definite steps toward recovery, that I'm able to understand how I used food and weight problems to hide from the real issues: relationship problems, loneliness, and shyness. Only when I took recovery as serious business was I able to understand that all of life does not revolve around fat or thin.

My weight stays within a five-pound range. I will admit that I would like to weigh about five pounds less, but I consider stopping bulimia much more important than being "thin."

This increase (eight pounds) was right after I stopped vomiting every day, but I have stayed at that weight ever since.

I am at peace with my body image. I learned the way I look doesn't count half as much as how I act and my attitude toward myself. I get more compliments on my appearance when I am feeling really good about myself than when I struggled to be thinner.

How should I choose a therapist?

Most bulimics should consider entering professional therapy. I'm often asked for referrals for therapists, and at one lecture, I recommended a psychiatrist who was considered a national expert on eating disorders. From the back of the room, a woman immediately cried out, "Oh no, that man is horrible." She went on to describe her experiences with him, which were indeed terrible. Yet I know that he has helped others. It is important to find the therapist that is right for you. Would you buy a car without a test drive? Some people spend an hour trying to decide which ice cream to pick in a supermarket. Choosing a therapist should certainly take more consideration than that. Put in time and effort to find a therapist that will help you.

Local health agencies usually provide lists of doctors and counselors who treat bulimia, and hospitals and medical clinics often have specialties in this area. Some hospitals that have inpatient units also have outpatient or day treatment programs, as well as groups available to the public. There are quite a few residential facilities devoted entirely to treating eating disorders. For some bulimics, hospitalization is an effective part of their treatment. (See the "Resources" section.)

As I've mentioned, there are different approaches to recovery. You must decide for yourself which approach best suits your needs. When you investigate therapy options, come with a list of questions. Does he or she emphasize the "abstinence" or "legalized" approach? Do they focus on changing thought patterns and expressing feelings? Do they give homework? How will they handle your anxiety level? Will they expect you to stop the bingeing right away, or allow you to improve at your own pace? How much experience do they have with this type of problem? Ask those questions which are important you to personally, remaining flexible enough to reevaluate your beliefs. Do what will work for you!

A "therapist" usually refers to a psychiatrist, psychologist, or marriage and family counselor, but can refer to other professionals, such as: licensed social workers, dieticians, or nutritionists. Also, some registered nurses, clergymen, acupuncturists, chiropractors, or those who practice therapeutic touch can provide invaluable services. A multidisciplinary approach combines several professionals as a treatment team. If drug therapy is a consideration, a qualified physician must be part of that team.

Check in the phone book and make some calls asking for references. Referrals are a good place to start, but you have to kick their tires! Call their offices and ask for a short appointment to meet them. Let them know that you are also interviewing other therapists—they'll appreciate your effort. Come prepared with a list of questions. This will not be a therapy session, so your questions can be hypothetical or direct—it's up to you. Some things you might ask are: What is their treatment approach to bulimia? How often would you need to see them? How quickly might you see results? How long would they expect therapy to last? What will the charges be and do they have a sliding fee, based upon income and need? Do they accept your insurance?

In evaluating the interviews, use criteria that are meaningful to you. These are subjective measures. Probably the most important area to consider is how you felt during the interviews. If you were comfortable with the therapist and felt that you could honestly work with him or her, that's a good indication. Other things to notice: Do you like the office? Does the staff seem friendly? Does the therapist answer you directly and invite you to express yourself?

Finally, you can always change therapists. Once you've picked out someone, try at least a few sessions. Give therapy a chance. You might decide together on a reasonable time period before evaluating your progress. If therapy with your first choice proves unsatisfactory, find someone else!

What can I do to help someone who has bulimia?

The support of a spouse, parent, sibling, or friend is one of the most valuable tools a person with an eating disorder can have. If someone close to you has bulimia, you can face it together in many different ways, but remember that they are the one with the problem. Loved ones can research treatment options, read appropriate books, attend lectures, talk to experts, and lend a supportive ear, but only the bulimic herself can do the work. (See Chapter Eight, "Advice for Loved Ones.")

Keep in mind that bulimia is a way to feel in control of one's life. Sometimes, what is intended to be helpful and considerate can be interpreted as controlling by the person with the disorder. Communicate that you are available to help, but that it is not your job to patrol their behavior. You are there to support and encourage them in their struggle to get well, but only if that is what they want.

Bulimia is a protective device used to handle pain. If it was easy to give up, the person would have done so already. Someone who uses food as a coping mechanism needs understanding and compassion. The reality of bulimia may shock or disgust you, but separate the individual from her binge-purge behavior. She deserves love and appreciation for who she is apart from the bulimia, and compassion for the pain that has driven her to it. If a loved-one became disabled or ill, you would still be there for them—bulimia is disabling and life-threatening.

At the same time, do not be manipulated or lied to for the sake of binges. Do not "enable" the disorder by looking the other way or pretending that the problem is not serious. If you stock the refrigerator with food only to have it flushed down the toilet, be honest and assertive about your rights and needs. Bulimics should not be allowed to abuse your trust or pocketbook; having bulimia is not justification for treating loved ones poorly. Also, don't turn meals into battles—food is not the issue.

Parents of bulimics especially need to be aware of their limitations in helping their children. Often, the relationship is too close for objective evaluation. Let your daughter open up to you with her feelings, and if she does not make progress with your support within a short time, encourage professional therapy. It may also be appropriate for parents to seek out professional advice or a support group for help with their own feelings of frustration and helplessness.

Parents usually play a part in the development of their child's behavior, and in many instances, may have to face issues and make adjustments of their own. This is not to say that they are the cause of the eating disorder, but rather that they may have contributed to it in some way and need to acknowledge that. Parents may need to reevaluate their values, ways of communicating, family rules about food, ways of handling feelings, parenting roles, and the family's decision-making process. Guilt, anger, frustration, denial, and cynicism are all likely sentiments.

As hard as this all sounds, family therapy has proved to be one of the most successful methods of overcoming eating disorders. With better communication, increased self-knowledge and mutual acceptance of what has happened in the past, parents and children can focus on the important task of recovery in the present.

What can be done to prevent eating disorders?

In the past twenty years, since I wrote the first publication in print about bulimia (Hall, 1980) and began working to increase education about eating disorders, I've come across hundreds of books written on the subject, countless newspaper and magazine articles, television programs, movies, radio talk shows, and public lectures. Numerous eating disorders organizations and treatment facilities have come in and out of existence, there have been informative conferences and workshops, and a whole new specialty has developed for health-care professionals. My efforts and those of other writers, speakers, organizers, therapists, administrators, and educators have helped real people. Also, due to increased public awareness, individuals with eating disorders are today able to find help more readily available and know that they are not alone with their problem.

Sadly, there are still millions of people who suffer with eating disorders and countless others who are preoccupied with weight and body dissatisfaction. In fact, after a brief rise and decline in the incidence of bulimia in the early '80s, which may have been due to the early public awareness of this condition, the prevalence of this eating disorder has not diminished despite our educational efforts. It is apparent that although we have defined bulimia and developed a variety of successful treatment programs for it and other eating problems, our long term goal must be to prevent these disorders altogether.

Healthy eating and the dangers of dieting must be incorporated into every elementary, junior high, and high school curriculum. We should further educate parents, prospective parents, teachers, the medical community, fitness instructors, physical educators, clergy, the media at large, and others about the symptoms, causes, and consequences of eating disorders, with early detection and intervention in mind. However, in order to be successful, prevention programs must go beyond the presentation of basic information, which has shown to be largely ineffective (Piran, 1998). Despite our best intentions, an hour lecture about bulimia, for example, may only teach listeners how to become bulimic!

For prevention to truly work, the approach must be participatory, systemic, and long-term. It is ineffective to solely teach a student about the hazards of eating disorders without also educating her teachers, parents, and peers. Too frequently, a health instructor will offer information on healthy eating and the futility of dieting, only to have the student attend a next class with a teacher who is on a diet, then have lunch with friends who only eat carrots and celery, return home to a family that is weight prejudiced, and look at magazines and television commercials that advocate the false promise of thinness. To actualize prevention, the message must permeate an individual's whole life; it must be integrated into all areas of our culture.

In a perfect world, free from eating disorders, all people would appreciate that love and self-esteem are their birthright regardless of shape or weight. Families, aware of the causes and consequences of eating disorders, would be a constant source of communication and sharing. Women would be safe from victimization in their homes, in the work place, on public streets, and in the media. Inner beauty and competence would be recognized and rewarded without regards to age, color, or body shape. Food would be a symbol of life rather than a tool for abuse. In other words, people would be allowed to be themselves without conforming to tight-fitting roles based on artificial limits.

There are so many different factors which contribute to an eating disorder that *all* contributing factors, whether they are cultural, social, biological, familial, emotional, sexual or other, must be addressed in order to achieve real prevention. This is a lofty goal that would require a revolution of contemporary thought. But I believe that every person who recovers from an eating disorder, every person who even embarks on recovery or who refuses to diet is just that—a revolutionary. And the repercussions of that person's actions can be far-reaching. Certainly, institutional change is crucial, but even those are made up of individuals capable of transformation.

Obviously, we have a long way to go, but we must each move in the right direction. Striving for far-reaching goals means that we must first face weight prejudice in our own lives and learn to embrace ourselves and others, regardless of differences. It is only within an atmosphere of mutual love and respect that we will fully realize eating disorders prevention on an individual, and ultimately a societal, level.

CHAPTER 2

Eat Without Fear

A True Story of the
Binge-Purge Syndrome

Introduction

I finished writing the story of my bulimia and recovery on my thirty-first birthday in 1980. I printed 100 copies of the 32-page booklet which I titled, *Eat Without Fear,* and finally felt completely free from bulimia. Getting it all down on paper was the final purge for me. What's more, I felt that I had accomplished something which could help others because, at that time, there were no other books solely about bulimia.

My bingeing and vomiting days may have been over, but my involvement with eating disorders as a "field" was just beginning. Those first 100 copies disappeared in a hurry, and I didn't even give them all to my family! The booklet was reprinted 14 times, making apparent the need for information and education about bulimia and other food problems. In partnership with my husband, Leigh Cohn, who coauthored *Eat Without Fear,* I decided to continue to write and speak about the seriousness of eating disorders. We have been doing it ever since.

This chapter, "Eat Without Fear" is an edited version of that original booklet. Including the various reprints, there have been more than 100,000 copies published. I've heard from thousands of people that my story has inspired them, and this edition seems as vital to me now as it did 20 years ago when I first wrote it. I hope it speaks to you.

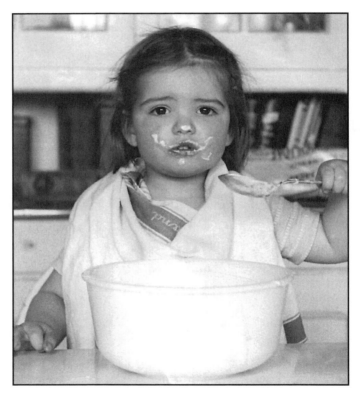

Lindsey Hall, age 3
(photo by LeMoyne Hall)

Beginning

I grew up in an affluent family that lived in a three-story colonial house an hour north of New York City. My father commuted to the city, where he worked as an investment banker. My mother ran the household. I had three older siblings who paid little attention to me—except for one sister who teased me unmercifully. Each of them was sent to a boarding school at the age of fourteen, after which I saw them primarily on vacations. I was seven when the fifth child was born, and my parents hired a live-in couple to take care of me and my baby brother.

The overall impression I have of my childhood is of being alone and afraid that I had done something wrong. I didn't mean to get in trouble; on the contrary, I always tried to be a perfect little girl. Nevertheless, I had the perception that I was constantly screwing up, like the time I put my sister's toy animals in a pillowcase to show to someone, not realizing they were delicate china and would break.

One of my biggest goof-ups was accidentally locking myself in my mother's clothes closet. She went to New York, and I stayed there all day, crying and afraid of the shoes which felt like snakes underneath me. No one heard my screams, not the housekeeper or my nanny, and I was not found until my mother came home late that afternoon. Even though I was rescued, I felt like life in that house could go on without me and no one would notice. I was not the smartest, prettiest, oldest, youngest, or a boy, any of which I believed would have given me some importance in the household.

I also clearly remember the atmosphere in our house, which can best be described as "tenuous." My father was easily angered and we all did our best to stay out of his way. At the dinner table, we listened to him tell stories of his day at work or joke about people he had met in the city, and wondered why he always sounded so much happier to be away from us. He sometimes put down my mother for not being interested enough in his work or smart enough to understand it. The older I got, the more this infuriated me, and I often stepped between them to deflect his verbal attacks.

My mother was a soft-spoken, well-educated woman who came from a large Catholic family. She was active in environmental causes, weekly tennis matches, and amateur photography. She had a darkroom built in the basement of the house, and I can remember spending hours with her in the dim light, watching the images emerge from the stinky pans of chemicals. I don't remember her losing her temper once, but then again, very few problems were ever discussed. From the time the nanny was hired, I spent less and less time with her.

Mostly I retreated alone to my room, attic playroom, or the empty barns. I had a few friends who lived nearby, but I avoided going to their houses for fear of their parents. One of the mothers used to laugh or yell at me when I didn't want to eat. Another threatened to hit me with a wooden spoon if I didn't sit at the table and finish my lunch. I was terrified of going there again— she made me eat tomatoes!

When I was ten, at an annual physical exam, I overheard the doctor tell my mother that I weighed too much. They said nothing to me, but after that I was conscious of my imperfect size. Salesgirls in the clothing store where my mother and I shopped for dancing-school dresses always sympathized with my "figure problem" and recommended "A-line" skirts. Despite my nickname at grammar school, "Thunder Thighs," I wasn't ugly or misshapen. By the age of thirteen, I weighed 135 pounds and was 5'5" tall. I was active, athletic, and actually had a shape similar to the one I have now.

I went away to a prestigious East Coast boarding school at age fourteen. Everyone else from my grammar school class went away to private schools too, for the local public school was considered "lower class." Without realizing how afraid I was or how to communicate my apprehensions, I left home in tears. For months I cried at the slightest provocation. I had never shared emotional issues with my parents or confided in friends. I didn't even know what was bothering me, really. All I knew was that I was desperately unhappy and felt terribly alone.

The other girls at school all seemed beautiful and distant: long fingernails, neat clothes, curly hair and THIN bodies. It was obvious that "thin was in" right from the start. I had heavy legs, which to me was the most disgusting form of being "overweight," and a small chest which was "undesirable" according to fashion. Having a pear-shaped body was an unspoken sin. From this point onward, I began to focus on my body as the source of my unhappiness, making every bite that went into my mouth a naughty and selfish indulgence, and becoming more and more disgusted with myself every day.

There were a few other girls whom I suspected had problems with food. One girl who roomed next to me was always buying quarts of ice cream and hiding in her room. Then she would proudly announce that she was starting a diet which required fasting for the first two days. Another girl lost so much weight that her muscles could no longer hold up her 5'10" frame, and she walked bent over with her emaciated pelvis tucked forward for balance. She was taken out of school with anorexia nervosa, rumored to have been throwing up to get skinny. That rumor was the first knowledge I had of someone forcibly vomiting. Even the other girl who attended the school from my hometown pulled a "crazy" act by eating hardly anything but oranges for several months. I visited her in the infirmary where she had been sent for blood sugar tests because her weight was so low, and I didn't know what to say. I secretly envied her willpower and her protruding ribs and felt like we had lost our friendship.

By the time I reached my senior year, my crying in public stopped, and I was no longer outwardly unhappy. I played sports, sang in the choir, and had one good friend. She knew I thought of myself as ugly, and often reassured me that looks didn't matter, but I honestly thought she was humoring me like my parents did. I avoided situations which would make me feel like a failure. I begged to be let out of honors math, refused to be nominated for any offices, rarely went to dances, and was afraid to talk in class. I was happy to get menstrual cramps once a month and retreat to the safety of the infirmary. I didn't seek out other friends, opting to spend my time alone or taking care of animals in the biology lab. I began to hoard food in the dorm refrigerator and sometimes hid in my closet during dinner hour, sneaking from my private stash of yogurt. I kept a five-pound can of peanut butter from which I sneaked teaspoonfuls when no one was around. Thoughts of food were often with me although I had not yet binged and purged.

I often tried on clothes in front of a full-length mirror to see if they had gotten looser or tighter. I compared my body to those of the models in magazines and the girls on diets at school. I feared I would never be thin enough. Who would want me? I took up smoking cigarettes in private, which in my mind was a bad thing to do, but it was better than eating. I chewed gum, sometimes up to five packs a day. Through all this, I managed to hold my weight steady.

While home on vacation at the end of my senior year, a grade school friend told me about a doctor who gave her a diet on which she lost ten pounds in one week. Playing down my desperation, I got my mother to take me to him. He gave me a pamphlet outlining the diet, and I returned to boarding school thinking that my life was really going to change; I was going to lose the extra twenty pounds that sat between me and happiness. I would be off to college, a new person, thin, confident, loved. But the diet was horrible.

I was instructed to drink two tablespoonfuls of vegetable oil before breakfast and dinner, eat only high protein foods, and drink 64 ounces of water daily. I lost eight pounds in one week, but felt bloated, nervous and depressed. Weak and sick, I went off the diet, feeling like a failure, sure that I would never be able to achieve what I thought was so important for a woman—a thin appearance. At that time I had a boyfriend, but when the diet failed, I quit seeing him. I also had the word "CHANGE" in two-foot letters cut out and pasted on one wall of my room, but I no longer expected that to happen.

I started snooping in other girls' rooms to look at their belongings. Kept on a small clothing allowance, I could not afford anything but essentials. I sometimes "stole" clothes, hoarding them for a few days or weeks until the newness wore off, and then I would try to return them, unnoticed. Often an item was reported lost and there was a big to-do about how low a person the thief must be, and I would have to maneuver the circumstances so it looked as if the victim had just misplaced the missing item. I didn't want to be thought of as a thief; I just wanted to be like everyone else for a short time.

The most devastating thoughts, though, were that other people could eat and I couldn't. I would watch the skinniest, most gorgeous girl spread brown sugar and butter on her toast every morning and never get fat, never even seem to feel guilty! What would it be like to live in a world like that, where you *didn't* think you were ugly? I began to withdraw from people and became jealous of everyone who was thinner.

The first time I thought of sticking my fingers down my throat was during the last week of school, after I saw a girl come out of the bathroom with her face all red and her eyes puffy. Even though her body was really shapely, she had always talked about her weight and how she should be dieting. I knew instantly what she had just done, and I graduated knowing that throwing up could be the solution to my "weight problem." Little did I know that my weight wasn't a problem. *How I felt about myself was the problem.*

I tried it three weeks later in a "Wimpyburger" stand in Oslo, Norway at the beginning of a summer exchange program. I remember the secrecy, the pain of trying, and the excitement that I had indeed found an answer to my prayers. I could be thin. I could be a success. I could be in control. I spent that summer living with a Swedish farming family. They were loving people, but I was unable to speak their language and felt isolated and unsure of myself. I was embarrassed to decline food at any of their five daily meals! I tried to throw up at least once a day, but, still experimenting with this dangerous behavior, I couldn't always get the food to come back up. My weight got higher and higher, and I returned to the States larger than I had ever been.

I shocked everyone—including myself—by being accepted to Stanford University, 3,000 miles from home, and I left in a blatant show of independence and bravery. Once alone in my single dorm room, however, faced with familiar feelings of loneliness and self-loathing, I retreated into eating to numb my anxiety and perfected the act of throwing up.

I began with breakfasts, which were served buffet-style on the main floor of the dorm, quickly learning which foods came up easily. When I woke in the morning, I often stuffed myself for half an hour and threw up before class. There were four stalls in the dorm bathroom, and I had to make sure no one caught me in the process. If it was too busy, I knew which restrooms on the way to class were likely to be empty. Sometimes one meal did not satisfy the cravings, so I began to buy extra food. I could eat an entire bag of cookies, half a dozen candy bars, and a quart of milk on top of a huge meal. Once a binge was under way, I did not stop until my stomach looked pregnant and I couldn't swallow one more time.

That was the beginning of nine years of obsessive eating and throwing up. I didn't tell anyone what I was doing and I didn't try to stop. I was more attached to being numb than I was to anything else, and, although falling in and out of love or other distractions lessened the cravings, I always returned to food.

I was convinced that bingeing was just a way to diet. Also, I didn't think there was anything wrong with it, even if I did it every day. I didn't connect my bizarre behavior with underlying issues, nor did I consider myself addicted, because I was sure I could stop anytime. Many times I promised myself that "this binge will be the last," and that I would magically, and with ease, metamorphose into a "normal" person as soon as I threw up "this one last time."

My letters home fluctuated between questioning why I was at college and vague complaints about my health. Letter after letter said the same things: "I'm afraid, but don't worry about me." "I'm sick, but I'm being brave and getting better." "I'm probably going through some phase." With every plea for attention, there was quick reassurance that I didn't need it; and, as much as I wanted them to ask me how it felt to be alone and scared, I would have denied those feelings. I know it. I was a smart girl, had been to the best schools, came from a family of bankers, lawyers, and Ph.D.s. I was athletic, seemingly independent and "together." How could I admit that I was throwing up to be thin?

Living with a Habit

I moved off campus my sophomore year because I couldn't stand the pressure of constantly being around people. I thought it looked like the kind of thing a "liberated woman" would do, and no one questioned me. I arranged my life to accommodate my habit, pretending to everyone, including myself, that I was being more of an adult. I vowed that when I got to a new place I would stop the eating and vomiting because I wouldn't have people around to make me nervous. I'd start an exercise program, become infused with willpower, get thin, and the world would be mine. The only hitch was that as soon as I was alone, the bingeing and purging took over once again.

I decided that what I really needed was a specific weight goal. I chose 110 pounds because I thought I'd look like a model at that weight. This goal stayed with me as an eight-year obsession, and I only reached it one day when I was thoroughly dehydrated from vomiting. Even then, at 110 pounds, my body image remained unchanged; I thought I looked the same—and that was fat. I felt the same way when I looked at myself in the mirror, too. Distant. Cold. Had I felt this kind of self-loathing when I was younger? What had happened to me?

If I bicycled home from school, I usually carried cookies and doughnuts to eat as I pedaled. Sometimes I got home and threw up that batch only to be overwhelmed with tension an hour later, and I would set off again for a frantic, uphill ride to the grocery store. Then I could glide home downhill, cramming cookies into my mouth the entire way, knowing that there would be full release once I got home.

Given a choice, I bought the same foods: one package of English muffins, a pound of butter, usually a package of frozen doughnuts, a bag of Vienna finger cookies, and always milk (preferably chocolate) or ice cream—and maybe five or six candy bars to start off the binge. Already eating in line, I told the checkers I was buying for a nursery school so they wouldn't suspect it was all for me. I could eat that much food in about an hour. If there was anything that I just couldn't finish, I threw it away, convinced and promising that this was the last time. If I hadn't bought enough food at the store, or if I was unable to get there, I would eat anything: a couple of omelets, a batch of sugar cookie dough, a loaf of toast, or bowlfuls of Cream of Wheat. It didn't matter.

Things were different now that I was living alone. There was no worrying if the bathroom would be empty or if anyone would think it strange that I came into my room with a grocery bag full of the same foods every day. The addiction was now in control.

I began to run out of money. My parents sent me tuition and a small allowance, and I was in a work/study program testing mentally retarded children. I was happy about the work because

I felt good helping others and the job kept me away from food for a few hours, but I always spent as much money as I earned.

It was at this point that I started stealing food. I felt a tremendous rush of success when I got away with a bag of cookies or pound of butter. It was similar to how I felt stealing at boarding school; I wanted what wasn't mine and what I felt was denied me. But there was one major difference: I did not plan on returning the goods. About six months later I was caught in a supermarket with a pint of substitute sugar in my purse, and the manager threatened me with jail. I promised to "go straight" and did, but the binges continued full force.

Marriage with a Secret Life

I had many short relationships that year which were fun, but not what I thought was the real thing. Then a friend of a friend, whose name was Doug, began to visit me. I liked being with him. As we spent more time together, I could tell that he was truly a good person. Talented, enthusiastic, smart, safe. Ashamed, I decided not to tell him about my eating habits because I was sure that they would be changing "tomorrow" anyway. I was twenty and it felt nice to be in love. Due to his military obligation, our two-year courtship was spent apart much of the time. When we were together for weekends, I would often be free from my food obsessions.

My parents loved Doug immediately, which made me feel that I had made the right choice. Picking him was at least one thing that I had done right! During visits home, however, the more he was included by my family, the more I retreated. They seemed to like him more than me. Used to feeling unnoticed, but not knowing how to deal with that feeling, I would eat. I felt and behaved like an outsider, sneaking my sandwiches and cookies, and throwing up in a bathroom with a fan so loud that no one could hear what I was doing.

When we left, it was always with the same feelings of disconnection that I had felt leaving years before. Clinging to the stability and safety of my relationship with Doug, marriage seemed like the logical next step. I didn't think it would matter that my mind was often elsewhere, dreaming about food, because on the surface I felt loved and in love.

For the five years we were married, the daily rituals and idiosyncrasies of my food problems became more and more rigid. I learned to put face powder on my eyes to hide the redness from the force of vomiting over a toilet, and on my knuckles where they became raw from rubbing against my teeth. I routinely ran water in the sink to drown out the sounds of throwing up. I stepped on the scale every time I passed the bathroom, as well as before and after every binge. I methodically tried on my clothes in front of a full-length mirror, hoping they would hang looser than the time before. I became a meticulous housekeeper, especially when I did not have a job and was "working" at home. Sometimes I delayed vomiting while I vacuumed and washed dishes, eating all the while, setting the stage for the "cleaning" of my body.

I was averaging three to five binges every day, which necessitated meticulously covering my tracks. Between binges, I ran to the store to restock the food. There were days when I had to re-bake batches of brownies a couple of times. I washed dishes constantly, and was careful to clean the toilet to be sure I'd left no traces. I wanted everything to be orderly and clean. The only thing that was not just perfect was me! And I was caught in a nightmare that I could tell no one.

Although we ate out a lot, I was nervous and preoccupied in restaurants. In nine years, I never ordered an entree because I was afraid I'd lose control. Instead, I would order side dishes, and suggest we get ice cream after dinner so that I would be able to get rid of anything I had eaten. I always ordered whole milk, because it was thick and smooth and made the food come up easier. I even knew which restaurants had private bathrooms.

To others I seemed like a health food freak. In public, I made sure that I ate only low-calorie, low-fat foods. I read books on nutrition and health, thinking they would be a positive influence. I took a course in anatomy and physiology because I thought that if I could see what I was doing to myself physically, maybe I would stop bingeing. At one point, I even took a course called "Creative Dreaming" by a woman named Patricia Garfield because I thought that maybe my dreams would reveal the key to my unhappiness. Little did I know.

I was surprisingly productive during those five years that my bulimia worsened. I finished my B.A. from Stanford, held two challenging jobs, and produced creative projects on my own. I started a business which is still running, and I maintained relationships with family and friends, albeit from a distance. But even though I was able to make my external life appear normal, internally I was walking an emotional tightrope. For the last five years, I ate and vomited several times each day. I could feel myself falling apart.

After nine years, some physical side-effects became worrisome. My vision was often blurry and I endured intense headaches. What used to be passing dizziness and weakness after purging became walking into doorjambs and exhaustion. My complexion deteriorated, and I was often constipated. I was usually dehydrated but didn't like to drink water because it made me feel bloated. Large blood blisters appeared in the back of my mouth from my fingernails. My teeth were a mess. Still, I refused to see that I had a serious problem even though the signs were obvious: a raving addiction, poor health, an increasingly distant marriage, isolation, low self-esteem, fits of depression, and secrets.

Shift in Focus

In spite of the intensity and secrecy of my bulimia, Doug and I did have many happy and loving times. We never openly questioned being together, but he was committed to many outside activities, and I had my food. When Doug got an offer for a fellowship at Cornell University, we did move back to the East Coast together, but he was often gone and I was alone to "do my thing."

As a surprise, in the middle of that winter, my father invited me to go with him to a small island in the West Indies for two weeks. Even though the idea made me extremely nervous, I jumped at it. Maybe chaining myself to a bathroom for nine years was beginning to get old. I don't exactly know. But I do know that I took a trip with my father, of whom I was deathly afraid, which began the journey of recovery for me. For the entire time I was there, I was completely free from the bulimia.

That in itself was a miracle, but on that trip something even more unexpected happened. In the middle of one night, I woke up and recorded in my dream journal, "I met a woman whose name was Gürze. She had mink hair and was inhabited by seven animals." In the morning, I reread this statement and looked at a drawing I had sketched of a funny little woman with long legs, a big head, and red heart-shaped lips. I didn't dwell on it at the time, and spent the last few days of my trip learning an unusual batik process taught by local artists.

When I came home, I began to experiment with batik designs, hammering together eight-foot frames for the fabric and spending hours over barrels of hot wax and dye. On a whim, though, I also created a five-foot tall doll, modeled after my dream woman, Gürze, and dressed her in my colorful batik fabrics. Then I made her a boyfriend, Dash, and eventually a whole group of friends, all about five feet tall and dressed as funny characters.

For a year I crammed my art between binges, and when I had accumulated a large enough body of work, I took my batiks and two of the dolls to New York City to sell. I planned to stay with relatives whom I didn't know very well, but I was determined to give it my best and scheduled appointments with designers. I tried to have enough confidence to accept criticism willingly, but the pressure felt overwhelming. Going back to the apartment was scary. On many evenings, I stopped at a market on the way to pick up huge stashes of food that I devoured in my room after everyone had gone to bed. One night, preoccupied by a binge, I left some important papers where I had stopped for pizza and ice cream. I ran back through dark, unfamiliar streets, oblivious to the danger. My food obsession had robbed me of rational thinking.

It was during this trip, though, that I happened upon a magazine article about people who had food problems similar to mine. This article was one of the very first ever written about the bingeing and vomiting cycle. The author, Marlene Boskind-White, considered what she termed "bulimarexia" to be related to anorexia nervosa, an illness characterized by self-starvation, but different because of the repetition of binges and purges. I was shocked! She was at Cornell, conducting therapy groups three miles from where I lived!

Also, incredible as it seemed to me at the time, on a Manhattan street corner, a gentleman inquired about the two dolls that were hanging out of my backpack. He subsequently bought them both. There was little interest in the batiks, but wherever I went people asked about the dolls.

My world suddenly shifted. Not only did my work feel turned upside down because people liked the dolls, but I couldn't get that article about bulimarexia out of my mind. When I returned home, I spent a week bingeing heavily and then called Dr. Boskind-White, who told me to come right over. On my way, I stopped to stick my finger down my throat for what I was afraid would be the last time. What if she cured me today? I wasn't ready!

During the interview, I downplayed my lack of control and the severity of the problem. This was the first time I had told anyone! I don't know if she guessed that I was holding back, but she invited me to join one of her ongoing therapy groups which would be meeting several days later. I told Doug that I had decided to deal with an old problem in a new way and added no details except that I was going for outside help. Far from relieved, I fretted at home about having to talk to a group of strangers about my binges.

When I got to the first meeting, I presented my usual false front of confidence, because I was embarrassed to admit that I abused food in such a weird way. I didn't want to admit exactly how often I binged, how much I ate, or that I was alone so much of the time—but I did. To say out loud, "I throw up five times a day," was extremely hard. But the women in the group were supportive and responsive even though each of them was struggling with her own food issues. All along I had thought that I was the only person who had such a bizarre relationship with food, but the group helped me see that I was not alone at all.

Dr. Boskind-White also stressed the importance of taking actions such as speaking up, honestly acknowledging feelings, and keeping a journal. I did begin a journal which I kept for several years, and just that small step made a big difference. I was learning to say in words what I had been saying with my bulimia. Gradually, I was able to put off binges for a day or two and I began to gain confidence that I would get better.

I attended five sessions when Doug transferred back to Stanford. Although recovering from bulimia was becoming my focus now, I was still afraid to tell him anything. Also, under the strain of my secret life and his dedication to graduate studies, our marriage had turned into a distant companionship. I decided that I should live alone for a while. I told Doug that I would return to California with him, but that I wanted my own place. I thought that I needed to change in order for us to be a better couple. This was my problem and I would return to him clean, pure, free, and independent when it was all behind me. He need never know.

When we got to California, we took separate places to live, which was painful and confusing for us both. We had never expected to be apart. Doug took an apartment in town, and I took a room in a house in the country. We saw each other practically daily, but it was always awkward. Even though I had started to undergo changes inside, when we were together I was unable to articulate or express them.

I liked Susan, the woman from whom I rented the room, and I hoped that I could open up to her. But I missed the safety of my support group and resumed bingeing almost immediately. Being around Stanford brought back memories, and I returned to the same markets and doughnut shops that I used to frequent. I maintained my journal, but I felt disgusted with my eating and wrote only about daily life, not how I felt. Even though I had taken some daring steps towards curing myself, I still clung to the magical promise of getting better "tomorrow."

An art fair in Los Angeles was coming up in two months and I decided to sell my batiks and dolls there. Even though I was running out of money, I continued overeating and vomiting, assuming that when the fair came, things would change. I would get to spend some happy time with Doug, who offered to drive me, sit in the warm southern California sun, and relax. But until that time, I stopped working on myself. Once again, my own well-being was not my priority, and I binged and purged heavily until the fair.

Turning Point

I'd hoped that the fair would be a turning point for me and it was, but not in any way I expected. Monetarily it was a bust, and I sold practically nothing. By the end of the third day, I was a bundle of nerves and broke down crying with Doug and his mother, with whom we were staying. I would not tell them that my greatest worries were about food, so they could not help me. I faced returning to my single room to my isolation, without a "real" job, unable to confide in anyone about the food problem that dominated my existence.

It was not these aspects, though, that made the trip a turning point. It was when I met a man named Leigh Cohn, who was also selling at the fair. I quickly felt able to relate to him, and we spent hours talking with each other when business was slow. I had never felt so comfortable with anyone; our conversations felt intimate right from the start—so different from my other relationships. I was conscious of his presence even when we were apart, and when the fair ended, only reluctantly did we say goodbye. We exchanged letters and phone calls as soon as we could and made plans to see each other a week later.

When he finally arrived at my door, the attraction was incredibly strong. For the next three weeks we spent almost every day together in what felt like a perfect union. Much to everyone's amazement, including our own, Leigh, who had taken a year's leave of absence from teaching, left his house, which was for sale in Los Angeles, to live with me in my room at Susan's.

Doug reacted with disbelief, and we had many confrontations right from the start. My parents had been upset by our separation, but they found it incomprehensible that I was living with a man I had known for only a month while still married. Even Susan disapproved. Everyone was against us, and I didn't blame them!

Still, I felt on a very deep level that for once I was doing the right thing, and I began to feel better in spite of the pressures. Unbelievably, the bulimia disappeared for those first few weeks. Leigh and I were together almost constantly and the sudden difference in my daily routine felt wonderfully healthy and refreshing. This seemed to be that magical, instantaneous cure I had always wanted.

As the days started to follow a routine, though, my newfound strength began to ebb away. I worried about the hurt I was causing my parents and Doug. I felt guilty for being so selfish. I was afraid I couldn't give up the bulimia. Who would I be without it? I began to question if I really was doing the right thing and if I knew my own mind. After all, I ate and vomited for nine years knowing full well I was doing something crazy; maybe I was still crazy!

Tension increasing, I began to sneak food while Leigh slept and when I was alone working at the studio I had rented. I could feel the desperation and loneliness building as it had in the past, and I was frustrated that being so in love hadn't completely cured me after all. I knew then that there would be no easy out. I had a lot of work ahead of me if I was ever going to overcome bulimia, and that if I didn't take the initiative right then and there, I risked slipping permanently back into the addiction. I wanted all aspects of my life to be as wonderful, loving, and free from bulimia as those first weeks with Leigh had been. The memories of the bulimia-free time with my father were fresh.

I decided to take a chance and tell Leigh everything—otherwise there was only secrecy and hiding. Now I wanted honesty and love.

Ending the Behavior

In a tearful, emotional outburst, I described my bingeing and vomiting. At first he didn't think it was a serious problem because he had never heard of bulimia. Besides, he had been a sweet-freak all his life, able to eat huge amounts of doughnuts and cookie dough without feeling guilty, gaining weight, or even getting cavities! His family loved big meals and boxes of candy, especially his mother. He assumed that I was just a sweet-freak, too, and threw up because I felt guilty about it. As I described the size and frequency of my binges, however, he could tell that something deeper was going on and that this was no ordinary problem. He listened with a lot of love and compassion and said that he would try to help me.

In the past, I expected to get better "tomorrow," "after this one last binge." But this time I knew that I had to start taking definite steps. I made two resolutions. I would be absolutely honest and tell Leigh about all binges, and I would do anything to recover—even admit myself to a sanitarium, if necessary. At that time, there were no treatment facilities specifically for eating disorders, and this promise conjured up scary, melodramatic images which I definitely wanted to avoid. Leigh promised to stick by me as long as I stayed committed to my recovery. He would help me come up with ideas about what actions I could take, listen, support, laugh, and love me; but we acknowledged that it was my responsibility to understand and overcome the behavior.

I went to see a psychiatrist primarily because of the tension and guilt I felt living with Leigh while still married to Doug. I didn't mention my bulimia at first, but when I did tell him, he recommended that I see a woman psychiatrist who had treated anorexics. I met with her once, but didn't feel comfortable. I realized the importance of confiding in someone, though, and decided to continue to use Leigh.

Without any guidelines to help us, we brainstormed recovery ideas. I began meditating regularly and recommitted to journal writing. I tried to establish a positive frame of mind by constantly watching what I was thinking and saying, and I consciously reframed negative "self-talk" to be more positive in my outlook. I wanted to feel more relaxed, so I took walks and listened to my favorite music. I decided to drink a set amount of water each day, but I had difficulty with that, so I revised my expectations rather than feel like a failure. Also, my doll business, which I named Gürze Designs, took off and required hours of concentrated sewing, during which I talked to myself about my recovery—sort of self-therapy!

I made lists: immediate goals, future goals, "Poor-Lindsey" and "Lucky-Lindsey" lists, what I liked and disliked about myself, reasons for wanting to get better, how I felt about my parents, my siblings, my life, ways to handle difficult feelings, and many others. I prepared a checklist of things I could do if I was on the verge of a binge, like exercising, sewing, gardening, soaking in a hot bath, and talking to Leigh or another friend about my feelings. Frequently I struggled, but increasingly I was able to overcome the urge to binge.

I had to approach food in a new way. In fact, it became my teacher because the way that I treated food was a lot like how I treated myself. If food was unimportant, expendable, not worth treating with kindness, then neither, I thought, was I. So, rather than labeling foods as "good" or "bad" which gave them power over me, I wanted to learn to eat anything without fear. I wanted out of any prison that existed for me. Toward that goal, I decided to allow myself one "forbidden" treat daily without guilt. This was a completely different orientation for me and was surprisingly easy. I began to treasure that one treat, which was a lot different than bingeing. I acquired likes and dislikes of certain foods and learned to say "no" by saying it to food. I began to pay attention to how I was eating and slowed myself down. Sometimes I had soothing music in the background during meals, and silently affirmed that eating in a healthy way was an act of loving kindness towards myself. This was fundamental, because I had treated myself so poorly for so long.

One unusual step I took had a tremendous impact on my confidence, but I would not have attempted it alone. *No one recovering from bulimia should attempt something like this without support and supervision.* What I did was to go on a planned, all-day binge with the intent of not vomiting. I wanted to know, at a deep level, that I could eat anything—that I could have power over food.

On the big day, Leigh and I woke up to a bag of malted milk balls on the bedside table to start. We bought a pound of candy, a dozen doughnuts, caramel apples, caramel corn, a batch of homemade cookies, brownies, and drinks—all to take with us while delivering dolls in San Francisco. During the course of the day, we also ate hamburgers and fries, milkshakes, a greasy meal of fish and chips, and continuously snacked on white chocolate.

By bedtime, we were both exhausted and stuffed. Leigh felt sick, but I was preoccupied by how my body looked and felt—pregnant and unable to lie down comfortably in any position. Leigh would not let me out of his sight for obvious reasons. I would never have tried this without a support person; undoubtedly, I would have vomited. In spite of stomach cramps, I was actually quite proud of myself at the end and laughed at what I had accomplished. This was a real turning point for me—I knew I could reach a goal, and I had power over food instead of food having power over me.

For many months, I ate mostly foods that I considered "safe," like yogurt and bananas or cottage cheese and pineapple juice, but I tried to stick to three meals a day with small snacks between. Eating that often seemed like a lot at first, but I was determined to stick to my plan even if I began to gain weight. Actually, I took a hammer to my scale after writing it a farewell note, so that I would not know what I weighed. Never again would I be ruled by a number.

I tried to change my ideas of what I thought I "should" eat to what my body actually craved by becoming aware of internal hunger cues which I had ignored for years. I started to try new foods. This was one of the hardest things that I had to do because I was so afraid of being out of control. What I discovered though, was that the more I restricted my eating to only specified foods, the more I wanted to binge. When I took the time to go within and discover what it was that I was really hungry for, I experienced satisfaction and fullness. Sometimes what I craved wasn't even food! Doing artwork, saying something that needed to be said, or just sitting quietly, was sometimes exactly what I needed.

Other times, I needed to scream into a pillow until I was hoarse or cry for hours on end. I released pent-up feelings, especially anger, by wrestling on a large foam mattress on the floor and exhausting fights with foam bats. We put on boxing gloves and Leigh let me hit him. He always pulled his punches, but came very close to my face several times. I took long saunas. All these things had a settling effect on my mind, too.

I began to explore spiritual issues because felt isolated from the church I had attended as a child. I read books on different religions and discovered many wonderful spiritual teachers whose lives inspired me to be more loving towards myself and others. Along these lines, I kept a picture of myself on my dresser with a candle and some flowers to remind myself that I was a good person, worth taking care of. I learned specific exercises which enabled me to see how my values and beliefs were influenced by my parents, my childhood, and the culture in which I lived. Taking all these things into account enabled me to discover the truth of my own heart so that I could live in accordance with who I was at the deepest level of my being. This was real nourishment.

The most difficult thing that I committed to do was to tell the truth all the time. I started by sharing my secrets about bulimia with the people I least wanted to. Doug, who had finally accepted our separation as permanent, was astounded, but took my finally confiding in him as an act of genuine caring. He said he didn't know why he hadn't asked me about spending so much time in the bathroom, and he was saddened by what I had gone through. Even though we were apart after that, I think we were closer than we had been in years.

About a month later, I began to write letters to people, permitting myself to send them or not. I wrote to my parents about how I felt when I was around them. I described my recovery, but did not ask for, expect, or receive much participation. I began to confide in friends, most of whom were interested, sympathetic, and supportive, though a few dropped out of my life. I wrote the following in a letter to my childhood friend, the one who had eaten all those oranges at boarding school: "Finally, I can tell people about eating and throwing up. Do you know how ashamed I have been all these years, thinking I was abnormal and disgusting?"

Gradually, I grew more comfortable with just being myself. I had always been desperate to maintain an image of unfailing perfection and independence, but now I stopped hiding my shyness, my opinions, my fears. As I grew to understand who I was and why, I also understood how well the bulimia had served me. It had been my friend, my buffer, my security, and my expression when I knew no other. It had been a way to anesthetize my overwhelming feelings, a vehicle for protesting my place in my family, and a place to hide when I didn't want to participate in life. As an addiction, though, it allowed no other behavior but itself and had completely consumed me. I fought hard to get me back!

During the first few months of recovery, I did binge many times, but these slips became less and less frequent until, after a year, they dwindled to one every couple of months. When I occasionally binged, I tried to consider it a way to learn instead of thinking of it as a setback. After all, Leigh and I had long talking and planning sessions after every slip. I gradually accepted that a single binge did not return me to square one. Instead, it was a red flag signaling that I needed to examine why I relapsed and what I could do the next time to intervene. This level of compassionate acceptance, coupled with a firm commitment, was just the approach I needed. The episodes stopped completely after about a year-and-a-half. It has been almost twenty years since I quit, and almost as many since I've even thought about bingeing or purging.

Lasting Recovery

Ending the binge-purge behavior was only one part of my recovery, because the bulimia had infiltrated all aspects of my life. Gradually, I have undergone a transformation in the way I view and experience every situation, from a simple conversation to a pressing crisis.

The most obvious change is in my relationship to food. I no longer eat to escape, nor am I obsessed about my weight. I recognize hunger signals and eat accordingly. There are no foods I avoid, and I enjoy everything from nutritious meals to decadent desserts. I stop when I am full, and feel no qualms about having seconds or leaving food on my plate. I do not follow rules and have given up my compulsive rituals. I take good care of my body and generally practice healthy standards. I do, indeed, eat without fear!

I came to realize that my eating disorder had less to do with food than it did with feelings. Instead of being numb all of the time, I now experience life in a completely different way. For the most part, my waking state is one of peace and personal trust, although I do get happy, nervous, proud, frustrated, satisfied, concerned, sad, etc! I have a full range of feelings, but mostly I try to maintain a state of love—my favorite.

Being free of bulimia has brought me in touch with an inner self I never knew existed. No one had told me that I had many of my own answers! This realization came from being honest and trusting my instincts. Once I made the commitment to practice honesty, I stopped worrying about what I thought others wanted and was able to focus on my own needs. As I learned to trust myself to make the best decisions, I discovered an inner self that would always lead me in the right direction. I came to respect and honor that inner self, to allow it expression in the world. It has guided everything I have done since.

As weird as it may sound, my bulimia is responsible for who and where I am today, because without such a serious illness I might never have worked so hard to be happy. I had to overcome every barrier that was in my way so that I could live and love fully, with my own set of values and ideals. From eating without fear, I learned to live without fear, and that has truly set me free.

In closing, here is a brief update. Leigh and I married shortly after my divorce from Doug, and having celebrated our 20th anniversary, we continue to be deeply in love with each other. Our sons, Neil and Charlie, have been great kids and a daily reminder of the importance of valuing children's individuality and contributions. As they have gotten older, we have kept our communication filled with mutual love and respect. My relationships with my parents and siblings improved, and I found it easy to make and keep friends once I stopped hiding! My soft sculpture dolls, born from the batik designs, were a rage in the late 70s and early 80s—nearly a half million dolls were sold.

Leigh and I co-wrote other books on recovery and self-esteem for our publishing company, Gürze Books, which specializes in books on eating disorders. Among them are *Self-Esteem Tools for Recovery* and *Full Lives: Women who have Freed Themselves from Food and Weight Obsession*. In 1998, I co-authored *Anorexia Nervosa: A Guide to Recovery* with Monika Ostroff, and Gürze Books has published numerous books by other authors. Some of our titles have been translated into such languages as Italian, French, Spanish, Japanese, and Chinese. Gürze is best known for *The Eating Disorders Resource Catalogue,* a mail order catalogue for books on food and weight issues, and we also publish a clinical newsletter, *The Eating Disorders Review.*

For years, I assumed that "Gürze" was a name I had invented in my dreams. But one day, about ten years after I had it, Leigh and I met a student of Bavarian dialects who claimed with great certainty that "Gürze" was similar to a greeting amongst peasants in a remote region of Bavaria, whose literal translation is, "Greet God" or "Hello, I see the God in You." This miraculous dream-name conveys exactly what I believe to be true. Every person has a source of love, or God, within themselves, if only they take the time to look. My recovery from bulimia was guided by this idea, and I hope yours is, too.

PART TWO

Overcoming Bulimia

CHAPTER 3

How to Start

The Decision to Stop

Bulimic thoughts and behaviors will continue indefinitely, and usually worsen, unless a decision is made to finally end them. I advocate choosing not to binge for many reasons: to live a longer, healthier, more loving life; have honest relationships; reach potentials of creativity; enjoy eating; experience peace of mind; save money; the list is endless. It does not really matter what your reasons are, though—what matters is that there is something you want *more than* bulimia; and, from that decision will spring your determination, courage, and willing attitude.

Some individuals have an easier time overcoming their eating disorder than others, but never is a cure instantaneous. Recovery from a disorder as complex as bulimia is a process of successes, setbacks, realizations, and resolutions unique to each individual and without a well-defined ending. Certainly, stopping the binge-purge behavior is important, but it is only a part of full recovery. The underlying causes for that behavior must be faced in order not to fall back on it in times of stress. This is an enormous task and one that is not to be taken lightly. Deciding to stop does not mean promising to get better "tomorrow," which is a bulimic thought, but rather doing whatever it takes right now to become free.

Even life-threatening behavior is hard to quit if it is serving to protect us from painful feelings, such as sadness, anxiety, boredom, spiritual emptiness, fear, or memories of a traumatic past. To give up that protection is scary; with little self-confidence or experience, we have no tools to face an uncertain future. Many bulimics just wait, wishing for a cure that will magically transform them without putting forth effort or work. Ultimately, however, they must make the decision to end the bulimia.

Everyone's reason for making that decision is unique to their circumstances, as these experiences indicate:

I've spent the last six months accumulating information on stopping my bulimia. But I've avoided doing anything concrete. Now hesitantly, shakily, I'm making a start.

Realizing that I am the only person who could stop my behavior helped me start my cure. It was all up to me.

Seventeen years is a long time to be in prison. I've done my time. I've earned my freedom. For me there are no concrete events or even attitudes in my cure, rather an existential decision in favor of life, which I continually affirm.

Really, it was the decision to stop that did it. Then, I had to be quite forgiving of myself and give up my need to be perfect. Eating better was contagious—the more I did it, the more I wanted to. It took me two years to stop the cravings.

*What has helped in my cure is seeking that cure. I became will-
ing to try anything to find the combination of things that worked
for me.*

Several bulimics mentioned that physical complications caused
them to question their behaviors. However, the mere knowledge
of side-effects did not guarantee that a bulimic would stop. Some
pointed out that they were "experts" on nutrition, health, and
psychology and understood on an intellectual level that their binge
eating was unhealthy, but still resisted making the commitment to
change. A nurse described her physical problems in quite specific
medical terms, yet hid this information from doctors who were
also her friends. A 38-year-old woman who spent thousands of
dollars on dental work during 15 years of vomiting felt fortunate
that the damage to her body was not worse. Twenty-two percent
of the bulimics that answered the survey were hospitalized for
their symptoms, such as these two who wrote:

*Fear! My emergency hospitalization for cardiac problems due to
low potassium was not premeditated or planned. Afterwards, I quit
"overnight" and never went back to vomiting, but it was very difficult psychologically.*

*An experience that made a big difference to me was a near-death
situation from poor physical health due to numerous daily bulimic episodes. I contracted malnutrition, double pneumonia, a
spastic colon, and hypoglycemia. I was finally hospitalized for
three weeks. Following my hospitalization, I got involved in an
eight-week group therapy, which met four days a week for six
hours daily!*

Pregnancy prompted some to stop because of a newfound respect for their bodies and love for their unborn children:

My bulimic/anorexic behavior has ceased almost entirely because I'm pregnant. I feel so much love for this baby that I want to love myself, too. A deep caring feeling toward others can sometimes set you on the road to recovery.

The experience that made the biggest difference in my cure was becoming pregnant and giving birth. The role of my body took on a new perspective. The externally-motivated desire to be thin— fitting into some societal prescription for beauty and happiness— was no longer in my reach. This gave me an opportunity to find or feel my own standards and to question "theirs" from my new, non-competitive, pregnant perspective.

I had a premature baby who lived three weeks. My doctors said my bulimic behavior prior to the pregnancy had nothing to do with the premature delivery. I'm sure, though, that fourteen years of bulimia, in one form or another, had a great deal of impact on my body's ability to handle pregnancy. I thought this experience would be enough to "cure me forever." However, about three weeks after he died, I returned to old habits. I am again pregnant and I do not want to lose this baby, so now I am eating normally.

Setting Reasonable Goals

One strategy that came up repeatedly was to work within a framework of success rather than failure. From this perspective, positive thoughts replaced negative ones, setback binges were opportunities to better understand the compulsion, and successes were rewarded with encouragement, positive feelings, and tangible results.

A woman who had read my original booklet, *Eat Without Fear,* wrote me a long letter in the early '80s. She had been anorexic and then bulimic for 12 of her 28 years. At first, she was relieved to read that someone else who was bulimic had "gotten well," and she went several days without bingeing. She opened up to her husband, who was supportive, and then entered professional therapy. By the time she contacted me, she had considered herself "cured" for several years. The following excerpt describes her early progress. Incidentally, we stayed in touch over the years, and now, nearly two decades later, she remains completely free from eating problems:

In the beginning, I had to make very deliberate decisions to do something else—to fight off an urge that I knew would only come back to haunt me. I had to accept that each time I decided not to throw up was an experience that I could add to my repertoire of getting better. This allowed me to accept any failures because they didn't subtract from my "getting better times." A failure did not mean all was lost. I could not throw up next time. I would use setbacks to examine the circumstances that led me to throw up, and from this I learned to avoid certain circumstances. I became more self-accepting, which enabled me to feel better about myself. I began to carefully examine how I felt after I had thrown up and also how I felt when I didn't. I gained greater trust in myself and in my ability to get well.

As I pointed out in Chapter One ("How long does it take to get better?"), recovery is an ongoing process. Of all the people who have shared their stories with me, in every case, recovery meant experimenting with different strategies and enduring pressures, falling off the horse of self-care and getting back on. Practically everyone participated in some bingeing in the early stages, but even those rare individuals who went "cold turkey," had to dig beneath the bulimic behavior to understand their emotions, causes for the bulimia, and triggers that set them off. Many shared that they tried to set reasonable goals, and some experimented with keeping simple contracts:

Basically, being willing to go through a whole hell of a lot of emotional pain and suffering has helped me the most. I make small, achievable goals rather than overwhelming ones. Gradually, I have gone from seven times a day to once or maybe twice a week.

I plan my day and stick to the schedule, not allowing myself to "play it by ear" and panic at the first moment I feel alone, hungry, or unoccupied. It isn't regimented, it's guided. I set small goals and achieve them. I use a checklist.

I'm trying not to be obsessed by the thought of an overnight cure. I know it takes time! Now I stop eating after less food than during previous binges—two bagels instead of six. My therapist calls it "discreet amounts." My binges have lessened greatly. They used to be my whole day, my whole life. Self-love really helps and also not giving up. There's always tomorrow.

I used to give myself stars for every day I completed without throwing up. I bought the shiny colored ones like I got in grade school. For some reason, this worked.

I put $5.00 in a jar for each binge-free day and saved up for something I wanted.

I stop myself from bingeing by recalling the pain I always experienced afterwards; and instead, I do something positive for myself, even when feeling depressed. Then I really "get into" feeling good about what I've done. This pattern took me a long time to get used to. I took baby steps the whole way!

Encouragement: Why Get Better?

The most important thing I can say about the struggle to end bulimia is that it is worth it. Even though it is more of a journey than a goal, and it begins in what feels like total darkness, there is a light that exists within your own self, which will guide you on your path to health and wholeness.

Surprisingly, many women who have recovered from an eating disorder believe that they are better off in the long run for having had one. They consider their problems with food and weight to have been their greatest teachers without which they might never have seriously questioned their beliefs and values or faced their inner fears. Recovery from an eating disorder made them strong enough to resist cultural pressures to be thin and to not judge other people based on their size or shape. They learned to respond to old patterns in new ways, enabling them to tackle other problems with confidence and compassion. They are often happy.

All these changes might be difficult to fathom when you are overwhelmed by compulsion and self-loathing, but remember that eating disorders are not just about food and eating. They are symptoms of inner emptiness and pain which, when healed, will transform the rest of your life. In time, you will find other things which will fill you up, not only physically, but emotionally and spiritually, as well. As one person wrote, "Self-love can be delicious."

Inside of you is a creative, worthwhile, loving person. In your heart, you know this is true. Stick to your commitment; continue to participate in life instead of bingeing. Practice love, and believe in yourself. Make lists, get support, enter therapy, follow our three-week program. It takes time for such a big change. Don't worry! Be willing to do anything to get better. In the words of one woman who wrote to me, "My life has not changed with recovery, it has begun!"

Every aspect of my life has changed. I now like myself. I am productive, confident, enjoy beautiful relationships with family and friends, intimacy to the max, my children. I am going through a divorce, and I'm happy about that, too!

Most of the time I'm fairly serene and better able to cope now that I'm no longer escaping through food. In some ways, life is also more painful though, because I must deal with the emotions instead of covering them up.

Since I have been completely free of bulimia, I sleep better, have more energy, and am less nervous and happier. I laugh more, and I'm told I'm more outgoing and fun to be with. I also have more money and more time to do the things I really enjoy.

I feel much more grown up, and that is wonderful. I am more confident. I don't avoid walking into a room of people. I approach each task with more strength. I enjoy little things. I am not so self-centered.

Physically I feel great. My hair is healthier. I just look and feel more attractive. I take better care of myself. I love my husband more. I am going back to college and I feel a lot happier and much more relaxed.

Suddenly, I have the time to get my work all done and play, too. I have much more money for hobbies. I'm settled now, happy, and eager for tomorrow.

It may sound terrible, but I was relieved when my bulimia was clinically diagnosed. It called attention to my other personal problems. Had it not been diagnosed, I probably would have continued to have difficulties with relationships, depression, and self-esteem. I am proud of the person I have become, and it is only because I sought help willingly and stayed with it long enough.

Although the my eating disorder had many negative aspects, I feel that without it, I would not be the person I am today. It gave me a reason to really discover my own truth.

I have ups and downs, like everyone else, but mostly my life is great! I experience happiness on a daily basis; I share love and humor and vulnerability with others. I never knew life could be this way, or that I could be this way. With recovery, I gained the self-confidence I never had.

I think I'm much more tolerant of others and their own difficulties than I would be otherwise. Also, I've become painfully and angrily aware of the ridiculous messages our culture passes on to young women. I literally fight these every day by offering opposing viewpoints to people who make shallow comments that seem to be accepted as the norm. I'm much more assertive than I used to be, and I feel more special and unique because of the increase in self-awareness that accompanied my recovery.

CHAPTER 4

Get Support!

The struggle to overcome eating disorders is much easier with outside support. This can come from many different sources: trained professionals, family members and friends, clergy, support groups, peer counselors, books, videos and tapes. When bulimics say that I am the first person they told, I always encourage them to seek out a "next" person to tell. One college student enlisted the support of everyone on her dormitory floor. She made a public statement about her problem and asked that they all help her to stop bingeing. They responded in full force!

Most bulimics are afraid that their husbands, lovers, parents, roommates, or others will catch them bingeing or vomiting. They are embarrassed by the truth, and think that being face down over a toilet is an accurate representation of their self-worth. Not only is the bulimia disgusting, but they believe they are disgusting for doing it. They are also afraid that they will displease others by admitting to such an all-consuming problem and be judged as less than perfect. Ultimately, they equate recovery with a loss of control and resulting weight gain, both of which are terrifying.

Unfortunately, this lack of trust, both in self and others, is the reason why many people are afraid to get support. Acknowledging the behavior to others means risking rejection, and if they have been hurt by someone close to them in the past, this risk may feel too big to take. Instead of allowing others into their lives, they develop resentments towards those people from whom they are hiding, withdrawing further into their obsession.

Being honest by giving up the secrecy and pretence is frightening, but a tremendous relief. Bingeing and purging takes a lot of energy, and so does keeping it secret! Remember that bulimia is not a reflection of the inner person, it is a way of coping with life. Unfortunately, it reinforces low self-esteem and creates a barrier to honest, loving relationships, as well.

Eighty-five percent of the bulimics surveyed acknowledged that secrecy was one of the most difficult obstacles to overcome, but their comments indicated the value of being honest and getting good support:

Coming out of the closet and talking to people has probably been most helpful.

A bulimic lifestyle is inundated with lies. Lying became so much a part of me, it was difficult to remember what was truth. I figured that if I told the truth and admitted my imperfection, I'd be in trouble. For me, breaking free meant always telling the truth and accepting myself like that—imperfect, but fully human.

I strongly urge telling family and friends about bulimia. It's difficult to conquer alone.

Telling my husband after four years of hiding has helped me the most. He is supportive, and I don't hate myself as much anymore because I'm not lying to him. Talking about it to family members and a therapist has helped a lot too.

Family Support

There's no denying that we are affected by our families in many and varied ways. When we leave home, we bring some of these attitudes and habits to our new environments. Whether you are living at home or not and choose to include your family in your recovery or not, it is important to recognize how they have influenced you, and to decide what to do about it.

An eating disorder does not exist only in the person who is suffering; *it is supported by the person's environment in some way.* So, in order for your parent to effectively support you, he or she must be willing to take a close look at the family "system" to see where problems lie. Perhaps there are difficulties with communication, expression of feelings, or problem solving. They might need to examine their own attitudes surrounding the same issues that you are facing—weight prejudice, women's roles, intimacy, spirituality, low self-esteem, getting needs met, etc! They might not be bingeing and purging, but they may share some of the same unhealthy attitudes that you do, which will not help you get well.

Also, parents serve as examples for coping skills and eating habits, and set standards for ambition, perfection, and acceptance. Although they may not mean to confuse or be dishonest, their actions may send conflicting statements. For example, a child may be told not to eat before dinner, yet may see mother sneaking spoonfuls as she cooks. Or, facing his daughter's coming of age, a father might withdraw precisely when she needs him the most.

An eating disorder is usually a way of handling feelings in a family where the expression of feelings is repressed, denied, or overlooked—especially feelings that are negative or difficult, such as anger, criticism, or defiance. There may be unspoken rules about who is permitted to get angry, when, and about what issues. Some families are unskilled at handling emotional conflicts or problems and would just as soon not hear about them. Children who grow up monitoring their feelings will find other, less direct ways to express them, such as with an eating disorder.

Parents also establish rules and myths. Some are direct, like no dessert unless you eat everything on your plate; girls should watch what they eat; or father always gets served first. Others are less obvious, like emotions should be expressed by yelling or silence; misbehavior is best disciplined authoritatively rather than with rational discussion; or boys can be trusted to stay out late, but girls are less responsible and must come home early. These myths and rules may have served a purpose when they were created, but they do not necessarily apply to your present life.

Overall, 91% of the bulimics surveyed felt that their families contributed to their eating disorder either directly or indirectly. Some were able to turn to their families for support, but others said that their families could not relate to food problems, because they either ate "normally" or were also obsessed. Meals were often scenes of confrontation or hidden pain and resentment. Many used bulimia as a way of getting back at their families. In any case, *the eating disorder was an added problem and in no way improved the relationships.*

Family therapy coupled with assertiveness training can be extremely helpful, especially when the person with bulimia is living at home. In some cases, therapists *require* that the family be treated as a whole. Ideally, all family members would share a commitment to improving their relationships. In this way, not only would the individual with bulimia feel supported, but the entire family dynamic would improve on a deep level, affecting every member in a positive way.

Whether you decide to involve your family in your recovery or not, it is still helpful to acknowledge and explore their influence. Here are some reflections:

Loved ones could not have helped me at all. I feel that my family was 95% of the cause. My mother and her entire family are obsessed with cooking, eating, and weight. The few times I have opened up to her, she has not been willing to understand, but just laughs the whole thing off and tells me I shouldn't worry about getting fat.

Moving away from my family helped, because I got away from their constant criticism and judgments. My parents always made me feel as though I wasn't really my own person, but rather a reflection of them. All of the neighbors and relatives would surely be watching to see how I turned out. Mom and Dad's success or failure would be judged, so I had to be perfect.

My bulimia has decreased almost 90% and I have my parents to thank for that. They have been very supportive and are always there when I need help.

I have difficulty getting support from my family, especially admitting to them that I need the help, and asking for it, since I have always been the one to help and support others.

The biggest help in my cure was the Sunday night reports I would give my mom. After an entire week without bingeing or purging, I told my mom about my accomplishment. I could see the relieved expression on her face, and that was enough to get me through any rough spots I encountered through the week. As each week went by, it became increasingly easier to not throw up. Whole days went by without even a thought of vomiting.

When I reached adolescence, my father seemed to avoid me, and I thought it was because of my weight. When I told my parents about my vomiting, he showed genuine love and concern. Having him involved in my life again helped me most of all.

I've been bulimic for 22 years and my family does not know. I am still afraid to tell them.

If you are a family member, do not coerce the bulimic into therapy with the belief that you are immune to counseling. You might play an active part in her history and recovery. Be ready to take a deep look at yourself and your own coping patterns.

There has been a vast improvement in how I regard my parents. Hatred is replaced by love and understanding on my part. More genuine affection is now shown by them. All of us are more honest.

Although many women described difficulty opening up to their husbands or lovers, the response they received was usually supportive and helpful. Most spouses do an excellent job! This also seems to be especially true of wives whose husbands are themselves eating disordered. I often get calls from these women, who are investigating recovery options for men reluctant to seek outside help. These examples are a small selection of many similar remarks:

The most important factor in my recovery has been the support of someone who loves me unconditionally, in spite of the ugliness of my problem. My husband now, boyfriend during many of the years of my bulimia, did not reject or leave me when he found out about my vomiting. He also never lectured me about giving it up. He did not, however, shield me from the truth of the physiological danger from my actions. In fact, he told me that I would most likely die from some direct or indirect effect of my bulimia if I did not give it up. The way he put it, though, made it clear that whether or not I chose to quit vomiting, I would be doing it mostly for my own benefit—although clearly he would benefit, too.

My lover helped me greatly by not being critical. Her feelings of love and acceptance took the pressure off. Telling her when I failed allowed me to deeply experience my sadness yet know I was still loved. She had faith in my ability to recover.

Professional Therapy

Most bulimics agree that talking about their food problems is extremely difficult, especially when they have maintained an appearance of competence and well-being for so long. While they may be embarrassed to "tell all" to a friend or family member, especially at the beginning of recovery, a professional therapist has no investment in seeing them as "perfect." Also, while there is a lot of self-help work that can be done on one's own, individuals with bulimia tend to hope that they "can do it all" themselves. This is rarely true and probably the result of a fear of relationships in general. Thus, therapy is a way to face difficult, painful issues as well as an opportunity to learn how to trust and interact with another person.

One feeling that a few individuals expressed was that no one other than a bulimic could truly understand the pain. Actually, many therapists specialize in this field because of their own experiences with food issues. But even if they haven't had an eating disorder, therapists are trained to listen, accept, challenge and provide coping skills. They are trained to fully "be there" for their clients, which is crucial for overcoming those feelings of loneliness and disgust which tend to perpetuate bulimia. A healthy, mutual therapeutic relationship will positively influence future relationships of all kinds. I strongly recommend that all bulimics seek out some form of professional therapy.

Many kinds of therapists and therapeutic strategies exist for treating eating disorders. "Therapist" is often used as a general term referring to psychiatrists, psychologists, or marriage and family counselors, as well as licensed clinical social workers. Additional professional support can come from dieticians and nutritionists, who can educate you about how your body works and prepare a food plan that is both tolerable and reasonable for you. Support can also come from school counselors, clergy members, and bodyworkers, who provide services such as therapeutic touch, massage, or acupuncture. No matter whom you choose for professional guidance, however, it is important to remember that their role is not to "cure" you but rather to empower you to help yourself.

Some treatment formats are: individual therapy, family therapy, group therapy specifically centered on bulimia, groups with various types of eating disorders or issues, inpatient or outpatient treatment, and halfway houses. Also, when individuals have a particularly hard time expressing their feelings in words, nonverbal, experiential formats, such as dance and movement, art, music, and drama therapy can be effective. Biofeedback training is an option for monitoring and helping modify the body's reaction to stress.

Although there is an endless list of topics that can be covered in therapy, treatment for an eating disorder generally revolves around three basic categories: the eating disorder behaviors, the thought processes that maintain those behaviors, and the emotions that underlie them. Cognitive behavioral therapy, which touches on all three, has been shown to be highly effective in treating bulimia by focusing on helping clients gain control over their eating behavior while at the same time lessening their concern over weight and shape.

Medication, or drug therapy, is also a form of support from which some individuals can benefit. These must be prescribed by a professional, such as a medical doctor or a psychiatrist, and are tailored to meet each person's needs. Be sure that you discuss with your doctor possible side-effects, the length of your initial trial, and possible dosage changes.

Of all the recovery strategies, professional therapy received the highest praise on the surveys. Eighty percent found it helpful, and it was rated "most help" much more often than any other category. The following comments represent the feelings of many other bulimics who also wrote about therapy:

Locating the right therapist for me was the most important element. Involvement in a self-help group was also valuable.

I saw many different therapists, from psychiatrists to non-credentialed counselors, but the last therapist I saw was the only one that helped me!

My therapist has helped me look at many aspects of myself of which I was either unconscious or that I had pushed aside because they were too painful for me to deal with.

Seeing my psychiatrist by myself, and at times with my mom, has been the best help to me.

I give my therapist a lot of credit. She never pushed me or put me down. She kept the attitude that I'd do it when I was ready.

The thing that has helped me the most is my group therapy. It enables me to see others with the same problem and is the only place I feel I can be honest.

One of my teachers recommended I go to the counseling center at school. This was the best move I could have made. My counselor has been very helpful in getting me to talk about my feelings and anxieties, which were being ignored or substituted for by my eating.

The most effective treatment which I have experienced was working with a team of a psychologist and a dietician. We began with a goal-driven plan, adding a new goal each week. Using this plan, I progressed from purging every time I ate to keeping down up to sixteen meals in a row!

Eating Disorders Treatment Centers

Many hospitals and clinics throughout the country have treatment programs that specialize in eating disorders. Typically, these centers offer both inpatient and outpatient services, and in some instances have residential programs, where patients stay in houses or dorm-like settings while undergoing treatment. Most treatment facilities employ a multidimensional approach using a team of skilled professionals, including: a medical director who is often certified in psychiatry, a program director, a psychologist who specializes in eating disorders, licensed clinical social workers or marriage and family counselors, a registered dietician, plus a well-rounded medical and nursing staff. Treatment can include individual and group therapy sessions, nutrition counseling, assertiveness training, relaxation and exercise programs, experiential therapies, and sometimes the use of medications.

Typically, the day will include therapy sessions, meetings with nutritionists, appointments with physicians, support groups, educational classes, and structured meals. Groups and classes may cover such areas as: body image, stress management, coping skills, nutrition education, relapse prevention, assertiveness training, art or music therapy, and expressive writing therapy. This kind of intensive approach to recovery is valuable whether you attend a center or devise a self-help program for yourself.

Regardless of where you live, there are probably some types of treatment centers nearby. Also, many general hospitals have eating disorders units. Consult your local hospitals to see what programs they offer, and for more information see the "Resources" chapter in this book.

Other Support

Support can be found in all different kinds of relationships. A few women from our survey described the value they placed on the unconditional love of pets, ranging from horses to dogs to fish! Others mentioned relief from depression and anxiety by walking in nature. In all cases, the support came from deep feelings of connection, which affirmed a sense of worthiness and self-esteem.

In addition to family members and professionals, good friends will be there for you if you ask. Seek help from teachers, spiritual advisors, and others who have recovered. Nowadays, it seems as though everyone knows somebody who once wrestled with an eating disorder and has gotten better. A recovered mentor can understand what you are going through and give you some insights into their own process. Ask around. Eating disorders organizations, local hospitals, colleges, high schools, and women's groups are good places to ask for referrals.

Free help can usually be found by contacting local college health or counseling centers which may have ongoing support groups. Hospitals and individual therapists sometimes sponsor free or low-cost groups that are open to the public. Chat rooms on the internet are another way of sharing ideas and successes. Another no-cost option is Overeaters Anonymous, a self-help group based on the twelve-step principles of Alcoholics Anonymous. One note: while OA can provide group support and encouragement, some of the principles which apply to alcohol and drug addiction may not be applicable to your recovery from eating disorders. We feel that different avenues work for different people. Take advantage of whatever works for you.

We stress that there is support out there if you look for it. We state this again and again, because making meaningful connections is so important, as these quotes indicate:

The biggest key I've found is expressing myself and reaching out to others for help. In talking with other bulimics and asking people to listen to me, I gain a sense of who I am, relief from anxiety and anger, and a secure feeling that I am okay. Today I have over seven months of no vomiting, part of which I believe is a spiritual miracle, and part is my willingness to show others who I really am.

The fact that most people close to me were not repulsed when I told them about my bulimia made a big difference.

I felt a lot less isolated after opening up and bearing my soul to two trusted girlfriends. Their prayers and undying support meant a lot. I learned that I was not unacceptable as a person, even if I did have an eating disorder I hated.

I had a friend call me every night and I would tell her how I did. Knowing I was going to talk to her helped me to make the decision earlier in the day not to throw up.

I encourage group support. Many heads together give different insights to problems.

A great decrease in my bulimic behavior occurred when I got a dog. The dog represented acceptance, companionship, something to love and care for, which was missing in my life. Gradually, I began to accept and care for myself, as well!

Talking to my friend, who was anorexic and bulimic for eight years and is recovered for three, is always helpful.

Any support group where people share their honest feelings is help-
ful. Isolation is the bulimic's greatest enemy.

Medical and Dental Examinations

If you are bulimic, your body has been through a terrible ordeal. For this reason, you should have a complete physical examination from a physician who is familiar with bulimia, and who will encourage you to begin caring for yourself.

The secretive nature of this addiction kept the medical profession in the dark for a long time. Fortunately, most doctors are now familiar with its symptoms and side-effects. Be sure yours is. If not, ask for a referral from a local treatment facility or therapist who specializes in eating disorders.

Sometimes doctors are intimidating because of their time constraints and implied stature. Be assertive. Do not make excuses to avoid a physical examination. Find someone with whom you feel comfortable and yet confident. The cost is no more than a few binges, and in most areas there are clinics available with sliding fees. Be sure to tell the doctor your complete bulimic history. It is important to be honest.

It is also important to have a dental checkup, especially if you vomit. Stomach acid removes tooth enamel, and constant exposure to food, especially simple carbohydrates, causes serious tooth and gum decay.

My teeth were an absolute mess for years and have cost me thou-
sands of dollars worth of dental work, but I have not had a single
cavity since I stopped bingeing.

I was afraid to go in for a checkup, but my therapist insisted. Finally, I went for an examination, terrified that I had every problem that I had read bulimics get. To my relief, I was okay, and that made me feel better about myself and my recovery.

I was a rock-bottom bulimic and was hospitalized with low potassium. The doctors couldn't believe I wasn't in a coma! As I lay in my bed hooked up to an IV, I decided that the bingeing and vomiting just wasn't worth it anymore.

I had to educate my family doctor about my bulimia.

My gynecologist found a benign tumor the size of a lemon attached to the base of my spine. She didn't say that it was caused by the bulimia, but I believe that it was.

CHAPTER 5

What Has Worked for Many

While we highly recommend getting professional help as part of your recovery process, we also feel that there is plenty of work that can be done on your own. This chapter provides suggestions for topics to explore, many of which come from individuals who have sent us letters and answered our surveys, and from therapists who specialize in this field. Think about how these topics relate to you, and concentrate on those which you feel will help you the most.

SECTIONS IN CHAPTER 5

Looking Beyond the Symptoms

Journal Writing

Practicing Self Esteem

Expressing Yourself

Relaxation

Working on Body Image

Healthy Physical Exercise

Experiencing Hungers and Feelings

Cultivating Relationships

Spiritual Pursuits

Changing Your Mind

Challenging Cultural Influences

Recovering from bulimia is no simple task. If you have chosen to embark on this journey, you will most likely be exploring unfamiliar and scary territory. Not only will you be investigating the origins of your problem, but you will be radically transforming your current behaviors. As uncomfortable as this may feel at first, think of it like starting any new venture, which becomes easier with time and rewarding on many different levels. Take baby steps if you need to.

We urge you to make recovering from bulimia the highest priority in your life. Even if you think you are being selfish by placing your recovery ahead of other commitments, remember that *all other aspects of your life will be enhanced by understanding and healing your relationship with food.*

Looking Beyond the Symptoms

There is a saying, "What you resist, persists." If you have an eating disorder, there is a strong possibility that you are resisting something in your life or within yourself which is manifesting itself through your behavior. It might be a trauma that happened a long time ago, a belief which causes low self esteem, unexpressed emotions, or something about your present circumstances which upsets you. Whatever it is, resisting the memory, the reality, or the feeling of it gives it life in some aspect of your bulimia.

In this way, bulimia is not just about food. Obviously, the immediate symptoms revolve around food, but bingeing and purging, planning meals, counting calories, and other habitual behaviors are ways of coping with other problems in your life. It is these underlying problems, which you are resisting, that fuel your bulimia. It is these hidden problems which you will need to explore in order to be completely free.

If you have not been able to stop bingeing and purging, looking at the other issues involved will help. Your bulimia is trying to tell you something, in a language all its own, and knowing this fact will take some of its power away. Your energy will no longer be wasted on trying to control your symptoms, but rather on exploring solutions. The bulimia has a function in your life, and your job is to find out what that function is.

Knowing the fact that there are underlying reasons for your bulimia does not condone it, nor should it diminish your motivation for change. Quite the opposite, realizing that you are using bulimia for a purpose can ease the guilt and self-loathing associated with the behaviors and make clear the fact that you do have fresh choices now, regardless of your past. Understanding the role that bulimia plays in your life is a way of getting to know yourself and ultimately care for the inner person you have been hiding. How has bulimia been taking care of you?

I just had my first consultation with a therapist and feel much calmer. My life has a new glow. Maybe it's because I feel nourished for once because she really listened to what I had to say.

I told my boyfriend that I didn't care if I gained ten pounds or not, I was going to prove to myself that I could be bulimia-free for two weeks. Guess what, I did! Instead of focusing on food, I focused on my thoughts and feelings and kept a journal every day. I learned so much and he supported me the whole way.

Write Your Story

Write the story of your life, with particular emphasis on events that are related to your bulimia, such as the first time you became self-conscious of your body. How did those events make you feel? When did your eating disorder begin? Explore in detail whatever comes to mind in order to get to know yourself and understand how bulimia has helped you cope. Perhaps draw a time line marking important events. You might also plot a family tree. Are there others in your family who have problems with food and weight, or related problems like depression, alcoholism, or social avoidance? Can you accept that your bulimia was a reasonable response to your experiences? Why are you pursuing recovery?

Note: This exercise can take days, months, or years as you get to know yourself better during the course of your recovery.

Journal Writing

Many people with eating disorders find it difficult to discuss their private thoughts and feelings, and a journal is a safe place to explore this inner life. They also have difficulty slowing down, because when they do, these thoughts and feelings become over-whelming. Writing in a journal is an excellent way not only to take quiet time, but to explore the issues that come up when that time is taken.

Writing is a form of intimacy because it necessitates having an honest, caring relationship with yourself. Giving your innermost thoughts and feelings tangible form makes them more real. A journal can reveal patterns that you might need to challenge, be used to chart your long-term progress, or help you problem-solve. A journal is like having a best friend who will always be there for you and value what you have to say. When you have the urge to binge, use your journal instead.

Buy a nice notebook or create a special place on your com-puter. If you are more comfortable speaking than writing, you can certainly use a tape recorder. Treat your journal with love and respect, because it is a representation of your own, inner experi-ence. Be spontaneous and let the words flow. No one else will read what you write, you won't be graded on content or gram-mar, and you don't have to explain yourself. You can be honest without being afraid. Schedule a block of time every day for writ-ing, and use your journal during times of stress as well as contem-plation. Consider keeping a dream journal as well.

If you do not know where to begin or get "writer's block," here are some topics to get you started. There are more through-out this chapter and in Chapter Nine, "A Three-Week Program to Stop Bingeing." Remember, there are no rules—write about what-ever is on your mind. Actually, by recording your thoughts, you literally take them *off* your mind!

TOPICS FOR WRITTEN EXPLORATION

• What happened in your life just before the bulimia began? Was there an incident that precipitated your first binge/purge episode?

• Make a list of ways you can fill up your life instead of with food, such as: nurturing relationships, self-respect, a new skill, etc.

• Pick a family member or friend and write your impressions of them, as well as describing your relationship. How has this person influenced you? What would you like to say to them that you haven't?

• Describe a particularly happy moment that makes you feel good just thinking about. Hold on to that feeling for the rest of the day.

• Write a non-judgmental, physical description of yourself. Next, write a non-judgmental description of your character. How do these differ from your usual, opinionated views of yourself?

• List ten people you admire (five you personally know and five you know from contemporary society or history). What attributes do they have that you admire? List your attributes. Which ones do you admire in yourself?

• Make a list of 5-10 myths and 5-10 rules that you want to change. A myth may be something like, "Skinny people are happier," and a rule might be, "If I eat dessert, I have to throw up."

• What can you do to become more self loving?

The following are more relevant topics to explore (Crisp, 1996):

MORE TOPICS . . .

- The meaning of my shape to me
- My family's use of avoidance to deal with conflict
- My use of avoidance to deal with conflict
- My relationship with authority
- My sense of self; social and sexual
- My impulses and the way I manage them
- My present or future career; why I have chosen it

When I began my recovery, I tried to make the journal my friend instead of the bulimia. In it I said whatever I wanted to say, knowing that it wouldn't judge or reject me.

I have kept detailed journals over the past 15 years. When I want to remember how distraught and obsessed I was, I read these. I am reminded of how far I have come, and how my desire for life, love, and happiness keeps me strong and clear.

I could always tell when there was something bothering me because I felt a twinge of anxiety right in the pit of my stomach. I always wondered if my bingeing wasn't directly connected to that physical sensation. Journaling helped me identify what I was anxious about before I began to binge.

Putting my thoughts and feelings down on paper made them seem more real. It helped me to feel less isolated, and I knew I'd eventually be able to communicate with people better.

Practicing Self Esteem

When you try to change who you are in order to conform to external standards, you constantly question whether you are doing a "good enough" job. Striving for unreasonable goals and comparing yourself to others turns you into your own harshest critic. You become alienated from yourself and feel empty inside. Bulimia is about this emptiness. It is a relentless, symbolic quest to "fill up" the empty place over and over again which, obviously, does not work.

The practice of self esteem is both a means to recovery and the goal. By getting to know and appreciate yourself, you can "feel full" with self-love! You are an important, worthwhile human being, a source of compassion, creativity, wisdom, contentment, and happiness. For some reason, which you will surely discover in the process of getting well, you have become cut off from this knowledge and don't even believe that it could be true. Without a foundation of self-awareness and self-love, however, nothing you do, buy, think, or eat will fill you up enough.

Therefore, the most important element to recovering from bulimia, or indeed any kind of personal "problem," is to raise your self esteem. This means developing a relationship with your own inner self based on the conviction that you deserve to have a happy life. In the past, you have thought poorly of yourself and what has it gotten you? An eating disorder! As one strong woman from our survey wrote, "I am a person, not a size!"

Self esteem is not something that magically happens. It is something to work at and practice, just like affirmations or writing. Get to know yourself. Learn how to listen to your inner voice. Be your own best friend by treating yourself with the characteristics that are important in a best friend: respect, honesty, trust, compassion, thoughtfulness, humor, sensitivity, understanding, forgiveness, and unconditional love. If you practice approaching yourself this way, these qualities will blossom in your life.

This transformation must occur on an intimately internal level. Concentrating on external change is futile. Being thinner will not make you feel better or improve your life. It may have given you fleeting feelings of self esteem, but more likely you continue to berate yourself for not being even thinner, more outgoing, or whatever you perceive you lack. However, none of these things matter, because what is most significant is how you feel about who you are inside. When you learn to recognize your own inner greatness, the size of your body will be insignificant.

The truth is that people come in all shapes, sizes, colors, aptitudes, interests, faiths, and so many different variables. There are infinite combinations, which makes every one of us unique. However, we are alike in that we all share one divine similarity: the source of self-love dwells inside of us.

All people have challenges and hardships in their lives. Stop putting yourself down for having such a strange illness, because even bulimia has served a purpose. Stop focusing on those things which you think you lack, for you are giving them life. Appreciate who you are instead of trying to be somehow "perfect." You are always a perfect *you*.

Repeating affirmations is a way to practice self esteem. Here are a few to get you started. Make the conscious effort to articulate at least one positive statement over and over throughout each day. Say it aloud, if possible, in front of a mirror first thing in the morning, while you get dressed, as you open and close doors, while you drive in a car or sit at a desk. Be kind to yourself by replacing negative self-talk with positive affirmations.

AFFIRMATIONS

- I deserve good things.
- My weight has nothing to do with my worth.
- I have a good heart.
- Every day, in every way, I'm getting better and better.
- The Universe is benevolent.
- My body is a temple.
- I am enthusiastic and confident.
- People like me.
- I am thankful for the lessons of recovery.
- I honor my individuality.

My value as a human being is not about my size.

My bulimia was a symptom of very poor self esteem, feelings of guilt, and helplessness. Through therapy I learned: how to treat myself with respect, that I control my own emotions, and to use frequent affirmations, which have turned my world around.

I have discovered at last how important I am as a person—a human that God created and loves. I realize that I am worthy of love and friendship; I deserve a good life, like everyone does.

As I became more comfortable with myself, I saw my life change in many ways. I found myself surrounded by friends who really liked me. And they were happy people, not miserable and depressed like my old friends. I have learned how to say "no" to people, and earned a lot of respect for doing so.

My self-concept has changed with recovery! I no longer have a secret life that I am utterly ashamed of! I no longer hate myself for continuing destructive behavior that does nothing but temporarily alleviate pain. I now love myself. I am a good person. Sometimes life is scary, but I can face it head-on now, instead of hiding in food.

I have found happiness. Once I stopped using food to cope with life, I started getting to know myself. To my delight, I like the person I discovered, and I now enjoy life.

I never dreamed I could like myself this much!

Expressing Yourself

Most experts agree that an eating disorder is a way to say something using the body that cannot be said in words. For example, expressing anger by stuffing food and violent purging may be easier than confronting someone who has hurt us. Even expressing simple opinions, if they are different from those of our family or friends, can cause enough anxiety to initiate a binge.

In order to give up using bulimia as a buffer, you must risk revealing who you really are and sharing your innermost self. You must stop trying to please others when it means devaluing your own needs. "No" is an acceptable answer if it reflects your real feelings. Be honest and be yourself. You are different from other people—everyone is—and that's the way it is meant to be! Here are suggestions for how to begin:

WAYS TO EXPRESS YOURSELF

• Think about what you say and how you say it, to yourself and others. Increase your use of the pronoun "I," and follow it up with active verbs such as feel, think, want, wish, am! Say "do" instead of "don't!"

• Stop thinking of yourself as "bulimic." You're "recovering from bulimia."

• Use positive self-talk. The mind can create problems or solutions depending on what you practice. Repeat phrases like, "I love myself," and "I am great!"

• Instead of swallowing your emotions, let them out. Try to determine what your bulimia is saying and express those feelings with words. Give it a voice.

• If you are angry, hit or kick a punching bag. Scream out loud.

• Draw, paint, dance, sing!

• If you need to confront someone and are not sure how to do it, rehearse with a sympathetic friend or in front of a mirror. Maybe write out what you'd like to say. Consider role-playing the conversation.

• Abandon your fears about talking to people. Be honest. Express your opinion!

• Seek out uplifting friends and support each other. Let family and friends get to know the real you.

I have gone from a person who went along with everything anyone else said or did, to someone who has and expresses opinions of her own and knows what she wants.

From the moment I first told my parents that I was "recovering" from bulimia, my whole perception about myself changed. I started to feel more in control of my own decisions.

I had always been told that I had no imagination. But in recovery, I started to paint portraits from photographs and discovered something that I love and am good at. My life has taken on an entirely new direction because more and more of the time I would rather paint than binge.

A large part of my recovery entailed letting my family know who I was. In the safety of family therapy, I told them that I needed it to be okay for me to be a quiet person even though they were all outgoing. It sounds so silly now, but at the time I needed to express that this bothered me every time we were together.

I discovered, and am actually pursuing, my own dreams.

Relaxation

People with eating disorders are under tremendous stress. Although bulimia can be somewhat calming in its mindless repetition and emotional distance, these effects do not last. In the long run, the constant pressure and overactivity of a food addiction adds stress to what already exists. One particularly negative consequence of this overactivity is that it disconnects you from your inner self and tricks you into thinking that you are only as good as your accomplishments. You then become a "human doing" who has to stay busy to be worthwhile, instead of a "human being" who is valuable solely because you are alive. Relaxation will slow you down enough for you to feel connected to yourself and your reasons for living. At the same time, it will allow your body to return to its natural, balanced state.

This is the magic of relaxation. Although you feel like you are doing nothing by being quiet, a great deal is actually occurring. Instead of being in the "fight or flight" mode, your vision, hearing, blood pressure, heart rate, breathing, and circulation return to normal. Instead of churning and spinning, your mind turns inward and rests. You feel more calm, more connected. And, when you return to your life, you are more relaxed, better able to handle not only the stresses of everyday life, but the challenges of recovery, as well.

For someone recovering from an eating disorder, though, relaxation can be quite difficult—even frightening. This is because, as we have said before, the constant activity associated with the bulimic cycle is a way of avoiding other issues, especially difficult feelings. Be aware that relaxation might allow some of these issues to surface, and try to let them exist without dwelling on them any more than the thoughts that pop in and out of your mind while you attempt to quiet it. Affirm your right to rest. Afterwards, cope with any of the "old stuff" that came up in new ways by talking to a friend or therapist, writing in your journal, or other strategy.

There are books and classes on some of the following suggestions:

RELAXATION TECHNIQUES

- Meditate.
- Observe silence.
- Listen to soothing music.
- Take a bath.
- Go for a walk.
- Stare at a body of water or a fire.
- Take up bird-watching.
- Practice yoga or T'ai Chi.
- Get a massage.
- Sit in a beautiful or holy place.
- Watch a bowl of fish, pet your cat, brush your dog.

Relaxation exercise:

Give yourself at least a fifteen or twenty minute slot of time. Comfortably sit or lie down in a peaceful spot. Gently close your eyes and remind yourself that you are a good person, deserving of great love and respect. Silently count to six as you inhale, again to six as you hold your breath, and once more as you exhale. Repeat this three times to slow down and focus your mind. Then repeat "I am," with each breath, and continue this until the time is passed. (You may substitute other words, prayers, or a mantra, for "I am," but it is helpful to maintain repetition.) Try not to be occupied by your thoughts, but allow them to pass through your mind and bring your repetition back in focus. If you have a problem or question in the forefront of your mind, make note and then go back to repetition. This takes practice, and there will be times when your mind will refuse to slow down, but eventually you will be able to enjoy a state of deep relaxation.

Note: This is one simple way to relax, and others are included later in the "Three-Week Program to Stop Bingeing."

When I felt sad, troubled, panicked, angry, or lonely, this disease jumped out on me like a Jack-in-a-Box. I just wanted to get numb! Taking quiet time made it easier for me to choose not to binge. I felt more connected with the part of me that wanted to get well.

I am thinking about taking some time off from school to find out what I really want to do with my life. I am so busy that I honestly don't know.

We have a hot tub in a cedar room with plants. I went in there last night, after feeling very stressed, lit some candles and climbed in. My mind goes a million miles a minute and I have a hard time with the relaxation stuff. My husband and I are going out to get some CD's, such as whales, the ocean, and rain, to help.

Sometimes during a relaxation session, I see a small ray of light and get a feeling of hope that inspires me to go on.

Working on Body Image

Sadly, the majority of women in our culture (and more men than ever before) are unhappy with their appearance. Our mothers, sisters and friends were dieting when we were young, and they are *still* worried about their weights. New weight loss programs and body sculpting techniques saturate the marketplace, the media and advertisers still primarily use thin, young models (although "plus size" models have recently begun to emerge), and fat women continue to be stereotyped as out-of-control and a plague on society. We have been so bombarded with the message that thinner is better that it is almost a revolutionary thought that we can feel at home in our bodies!

This discontent goes deeper than the surface, though, because how we feel about our bodies is closely aligned with our self image. The two go hand in hand. For this reason, no matter how good conforming to an external ideal might make you feel, you won't truly like your outer self until you like your inner self. Other people can even tell you that you are beautiful, but unless you feel self-love, you will be dissatisfied with your body.

I am sure that we have said, but it is worth repeating, that bodies come in all shapes and sizes and you have been born with a certain body type that you can find somewhere on your family tree. Your natural size can be altered to some degree by the food you eat and the amount of exercise you get, but you cannot radically change your inherited body type without harming yourself through obsessive exercise, surgery, or an eating disorder. However, as you already know, the rewards of such excesses do not materialize. Ask yourself: Has obsessing about thinness brought you the loving relationships, satisfying jobs, and meaningful successes that you expected?

Although it might seem so, disliking your body isn't part of the female condition. It is a learned response to a culture that glorifies thinness. Weight prejudice is the most socially-accepted form of hatred we know. Author W. Charisse Goodman exposes this bigotry in her book, *The Invisible Woman: Confronting Weight Prejudice in America:*

"A big woman is neither seen nor heard in our thinness-ob-sessed society, and is defined purely in terms of her weight and other people's prejudice. Regardless of her unique per-sonal qualities, she is faced with images which portray her as an unattractive, sloppy, even anti-social type. Whatever her in-dividual health habits may be, she must cope with a popular attitude that insists she is compulsive, self-indulgent, sick, and lazy. No matter how well-loved or loving she may be, she con-stantly gets the message that she is hiding from intimate rela-tionships behind her full flesh." (1995)

Your recovery from bulimia in part depends on your ability to accept your body, as well as the bodies of all people. Self worth is not a size. Your body is neither good nor bad, it is just the one you inherited. Consider the possibility that there is no such thing as an ideal body, and that phrases like, "I feel fat," and, "I look ugly," are indications that there is something else bothering you that goes beyond the way you look. Making disparaging remarks about your body is as addictive as bingeing, and just like binge-ing, is an indication of underlying issues. You have to defy cul-tural influences and love your body. You have to be a revolutionary!

You can do many things to improve how you feel about your body. Here are some ideas:

SUGGESTIONS FOR IMPROVING BODY IMAGE

- Smile more, look happier.

- Walk and speak with dignity. Let your body lan-guage reflect this emerging pride.

- Go to a dance or yoga class and leave your inhibitions at home.

- Use affirmations to change negative self-talk.

- Try guided imagery and visualization techniques to support self-acceptance and to handle fears associated with body changes.

- Make friends with some large men or women.

- Notice that everyone's body is different and stop comparing yourself. Neither ultra-thin models nor the super heavy should be judged by their bodies, and neither should you.

- Practice movement exercises to reacquaint yourself with how your body feels.

- Appreciate your sexuality. Have an orgasm!

- Thank your body for all the good things it does for you. Pamper it with massages and warm baths.

- Take a couple of days off for a personal vacation during your menstruation.

- Get moderate daily exercise.

- Buy clothes that fit.

- Stop looking in the mirror so often and judging specific parts of your body. See the whole.

- Throw out—or destroy—your scale.

- Accept compliments graciously, knowing that beauty on the outside reflects the beauty on the inside.

- Read books on improving body image.

Visualization exercise

Get settled and close your eyes in a quiet, comfortable place. After a few cleansing breaths, imagine yourself as a toddler. See how round you are as you roll on the floor or pull yourself up to stand. Hear the adults saying, "What a darling child." Feel happiness in knowing that they are talking about you. The fat on the child is okay, because it is natural for all children to have baby fat. Then, picture yourself as a young teenager, just starting to mature. Your body needs to grow at this time; it needs some extra fat, too. Now, see yourself moving into adulthood, getting some wrinkles and letting gravity take over a bit. Can you accept these changes? Finally, imagine yourself at 90 years old. How far your body has taken you! What do you look like? How do you feel towards your body now? Bodies change. Relax. Get comfortable with this idea and appreciate what nature gave you.

I like my body! And, it is 10-12 pounds heavier than I thought I could live with.

I didn't see my body the way others did. The difference now is that I acknowledge my perceptions to be distorted by my low self esteem, and let it sit at that. I recognize that I didn't "feel thin" at 85 pounds, so losing weight is not my answer anymore.

My physical body is a map, a reflection of the totality of every experience I have had since conception, and the genetic disposition of my family of origin. It is unique like I am.

My body image is based on my feelings about myself at that moment. In other words, how I see myself is based on my emotions.

More and more now, I have times when I am at peace with my body image because I feel more at peace internally. I am glad I am healthy and not emaciated, as I used to be.

Most of my life I have used my body size to evaluate my self-worth. It wasn't until my mid-forties that I finally began to recognize that others valued me for who I was, not how I looked.

Healthy Physical Exercise

Exercise is a wonderful way to enhance our feelings of well-being and general health, but there is a difference between healthy moderate exercise and working out obsessively. For someone with an eating disorder, exercise can be a type of purge. While it may be healthy to jog 10-15 miles per week, running that many miles per day goes far beyond the scope of merely staying fit.

Some researchers claim that chemical changes within the body cause an addictive exercise "high" which is not necessarily harmful. While this may be true, excessive exercise can a be a way to: purge unwanted calories, (seemingly) regain the control that was lost during a binge, release overwhelming emotions, or escape responsibilities or difficult issues. Extreme training can masquerade as a fitness regime and trick us into thinking we are being good to ourselves when we most certainly are not.

On the other hand, healthy exercise is an important part of a multidimensional, self-nurturing program. Healthy people enjoy regular exercise, and more than 80% of the recovered bulimics we surveyed found it extremely satisfying, mentally, emotionally, and physically. When you exercise, you feel good—unless you are obsessive and compulsive about it.

We do not suggest one form of exercise over another. Team sports or group activities are just as helpful as working out by yourself, and there is a lot to be gained by being with others. Walk with a friend! Twenty or forty minutes of vigorous activity up to six days per week is reasonable, and you can supplement that with other, less aerobic movement, stretching, strengthening, yoga, etc.

To get the most out of your workout, we stress the importance of a positive attitude, stretching (see the short guide to stretching on Day One of "A Three-Week Program to Stop Bingeing"), and allowing yourself time to relax and reflect afterwards. Take advantage of all the good feelings that come from moving your body!

RECOMMENDED ACTIVITIES

Aerobic Workouts
- Jogging
- Biking
- Swimming
- In-line skating
- Hiking
- Fast walking
- Basketball
- Tennis
- Racquetball
- Volleyball
- Stairmaster

- Jumping rope
- Cross country skiing
- Surfing
- Rowing
- Vigorous dance
- Martial arts

Supplemental Activities

- Weight training
- Yoga
- Golf
- Bowling
- Gardening
- Group or partner dancing
- Leisure walking

I've found exercise to be very helpful. Afterwards, I'll tend to eat normally instead of my usual cram session. I jog, but I suppose any type of exercise that works up a good, honest sweat will do!

To help ease anxiety and frustration, I swim or bike ride. This releases a lot of built-up energy that I usually use for a binge; bingeing is exhausting! After exercising I feel so much better about myself. I'm proud because I chose to do something good for me instead of destructively bingeing.

I used to compulsively jog five miles a day and work out at the gym. Sometimes I hadn't eaten in a long time and felt dizzy and weak. When I started to recover, it was hard to normalize both patterns at the same time, so first I quit exercising altogether and just concentrated on my fear of food. After I was able to tolerate feeding myself fairly well, I added walking, and now swim or jog a few times a week. I'm really doing well.

Daily exercise is essential for my mental, emotional, physical, and spiritual health. I try to do some aerobics every day, walk, swim, bike, etc. But if I miss a day, that's okay too.

Exercise makes me feel good, look better, and sleep great. It helps me have more energy, makes me feel strong, and eases stress.

Experiencing Hungers and Feelings

Human beings have various types of hungers—physical, emotional, social, spiritual, and sexual, among others. People with eating disorders have difficulty recognizing the differences, because they are separated from their inner experience by an addiction to binges and purges. Therefore, an important aspect of recovery is to gently let go of the behaviors long enough to distinguish between these hungers—especially the physical and emotional ones—and to feed them appropriately.

Physical hunger is our body's physiological craving for nourishment. Emotional hunger is a complex mix of needs, desires and feelings. Being unable or unwilling to face these inner issues, a bulimic will respond in a symbolic way by eating until they can literally hold no more food; but all of the food in the world cannot satisfy emotional needs.

Typically, bulimics are propelled into binges by what they would describe as overwhelming feelings of anxiety, like a "mass" of emotional pressure. Food, and the act of getting it down as quickly as possible, is a distraction from this anxiety and often a way of avoiding it altogether. But if you are on the road to recovery, you will need to stop and ask yourself *before* the binge begins, "What am I truly hungry for? What feelings need to be expressed? Is there a way of satisfying my hungers directly instead of routing them through bulimia?" Be gentle and compassionate with yourself as you attempt to stop your binges and allow your feelings to surface, knowing that there might be pain or fear underneath. Get support with this difficult challenge.

Every binge is a teacher because it gives us the opportunity to learn more about ourselves and why we are abusing food. Each of us has a rich and powerful inner life, and to deny it is to deny a part of ourselves. Emotional hungers are legitimate and need to be satisfied in appropriate ways. For example, if you are worried about a relationship, instead of bingeing, discuss your concerns with the other person or write about them. If you feel lonely, instead of spending time alone eating, call a friend, attend a class, or join a support group. If you are anxious about money, talk to a financial counselor or look into getting a better job. The point is to experience your emotions instead of burying them with food. Remember, no amount of eating will satisfy emotional hunger.

For someone who has been bulimic for a number of years, physical hunger signals can be extremely difficult to recognize. Some recovering bulimics respond well to food plans, which remove the responsibility for choosing when and how much to eat. These can be particularly helpful in the early stages of recovery, when emotional hungers are surfacing and you are more tempted to succumb to old coping habits. Others choose to "legalize" foods and ease restrictions in an attempt to experience their hunger cues as they naturally occur. (See Chapter Six "Healthy Eating & Healthy Weight.")

I feel best about myself when I eat in response to physical hunger. This feels like I am honoring my inner self. To eat in response to emotional hunger, without the presence of the physical, is my definition of compulsive eating.

I used to binge when I was upset, bored, or anxious. Now, I think about my feelings and try to find alternate things to do.

I am learning through self-awareness and therapy that I have often chosen to eat rather than feel anxiety and anger. I am now able to express my anger and sit with anxiety. I understand that feelings pass and that I can choose not to eat.

Being terribly abused by the man I loved was the precursor to my bulimia. I binged to stuff the hurt and fill the void. Now, I am filled with love, but it comes from within me, not from someone else.

Without realizing it, I substituted food for many emotions. In my recovery, I'm learning to recognize that my sudden hunger or cravings are actually emotions or signs of something bothering me.

Cultivating Relationships

Secrecy and isolation are part of a bulimic's lifestyle because their primary relationship is with food, rather than with themselves or other people. Therefore, it should come as no surprise that recovery means breaking down the barriers to intimacy and learning how to develop healthy, caring relationships.

Finding people to confide in is crucial, especially for someone whose boundaries are unclear or who has been hurt in the past. Therapists are good choices because they know how to guide, teach, challenge, and be there for you when needed. A willing friend or relative can be a safe sounding board. Help can also be found in support groups with people who have faced or are facing similar problems. The important thing is to interact with others who will mirror your earnest effort to love and be loved. Gradually and gently, allow more people to know who you really are. You might be amazed at how supportive some can be. Eventually, you will become more and more comfortable with who you are, and be able to maintain that sense of self even as you connect with others.

As you gather the confidence to express your thoughts, feelings, and needs, you will be able to tackle relationships with some of the more difficult people in your life. Be aware of old, restrictive roles, and especially do not allow yourself to be abused. Separation and independence is a better choice than being misunderstood or mistreated. Also, if you have low self esteem, you probably tend to have superficial "friendships" with others who also have low self esteem. You don't need people who bring you down when you are sincerely working on your recovery. Develop positive relationships with those who want to be uplifting and self-accepting. Keep good company! This is so important, I will repeat it for you: Keep good company!

Additionally, you may need to address issues regarding your sexuality. Sometimes bulimia is used to avoid the intimacy of sexual relationships in response to sexual victimization, ranging from rape to the objectification of women in a male-dominated society. It is a way to have predictable physical pleasure alone. Gorging and purging is similar to the act and feelings of sexual intercourse—the slow buildup of intensity, the emotional craving for love, the stroking of the body, the explosion of physical pleasure/pain, and for some, a conditioned guilt. However, recovery creates the opportunity for having all kinds of love in your life. As you increase your self esteem and your capacity for intimacy, you will be more ready and capable of having satisfying sexual relationships as well.

People with bulimia are afraid of relationships. Their guilt and secrecy cause them to fear what people think of them. But everyone has some fear about exposing their true selves to the outside world, and your recovery can be helped by becoming open and honest with select other people. Giving up bulimia as a "best friend" means rediscovering friendship and intimacy, which requires courage and practice. Here are a few suggestions:

IDEAS FOR CULTIVATING HEALTHY RELATIONSHIPS

- Be honest at all times.
- Reach out to long distance friends with letters, calls, and e-mail.
- Seek out a long-lost friend who knew and liked you before you had bulimia.
- If you anticipate a conversation to be difficult or confrontational, try role playing it first with a friend or therapist.
- Make eye contact.

- Smile, laugh, have fun!
- Volunteer at a retirement home and "adopt" someone who is lonely.
- Spend time with small children or animals—they accept you unconditionally.
- Assert yourself; say what's on your mind.
- Be positive.
- Ask questions, listen, and be supportive.
- Keep good company!
- See God in everyone, especially yourself.

Because most of us who have bulimia are ashamed of our behavior, we tend to hide and keep our addiction a secret. We isolate from the ones who care and want to help us. There were many times I wanted to go to someone for help, but fear of rejection kept me isolated. I can't tell you what a relief it was when my secret was finally out in the open—everyone who knows has been very supportive and understanding.

My saving grace has been your book and my sister, who is a recovered anorexic. I've debated telling my best friend who will be at college with me next year but I know unless I do, the relationship won't be honest and we will grow apart.

I think maybe initially I was getting better for my husband and hoped that eventually I would want to get better for me. This is exactly what has happened. When I was honest, our relationship deepened, and I discovered that I was a good person. That gave me confidence. Now I have a close girlfriend and generally feel more comfortable around other people.

Eating can be very sexual. I'm sure it's not a coincidence, but I never had an orgasm until I stopped purging. Purging was almost a type of oral masturbation.

I found it a real challenge to let my friends know about my problem. Thinking of their reactions was scary, but as long as I kept my secret, I couldn't get close to them. It seemed like I had everything— good grades, lots of dates. Little did they know that inside I was feeling inadequate, insecure and suffering from low self esteem. I felt so stressed that I gradually began to pull myself back, leaving myself lonely to binge and purge in peace. In my recovery process, I started to socialize again, and this time I chose a couple of friends who I thought I could trust with my secret. Their reactions were the very opposite of what I had feared—they were understanding and supportive, offering to help me in any way they could. I was so relieved. Their acceptance gave me more confidence and made it easier for me to tell other people. Not everyone had the same caring response, but I was able to accept that. I have no regrets about telling anyone. In fact, one of my closest, lifelong friends shared that she was suffering from the same disease. We were able to be there for one another in a way we had never been before.

Spiritual Pursuits

Eating disorders are about feeling empty inside, not just physically or emotionally, but spiritually as well. They are tools for coping with a life which lacks love, meaning, a sense of safety, connections to others, and self esteem. Exploring these areas is what I call "spiritual pursuit" or recognizing the spirit that dwells within ourselves and everyone, apart from our minds and bodies. This spirit is called many names, such as: God, Higher Power, the Self, collective unconscious, etc. Tending to the health of our spirit connects us to the mystery of life and satisfies us at a level we do not completely comprehend.

The most fulfilling thing I have done throughout my recovery has been to practice love. This has been my path—loving myself and loving others. This simple teaching forced me to look at the barriers I had to experiencing love in all areas of my life, which was the thing that I was most hungry for. I'm not talking solely about the love for my husband or children, but rather a pervasive state of love with which I could approach every person, place, and situation. Being on this spiritual path has given my life meaning and satisfied me in a way food never did. Ironically, I have my bulimia to thank for it! As we wrote in our book, *Self Esteem Tools for Recovery*,

> "When we practice love, we are making a connection with our real selves. This love cuts through the layers of false selves that we wear for protection, and makes clear that we are at our core, not flawed, but divine. We come in contact with our capacity for compassion, creativity, humor, goodness, and love. We realize that we are truly worthy of self esteem."

In recent years, more and more therapists are integrating spirituality into their treatment of eating disorders, as therapist Carolyn Costin explains,

"I have come to view my treatment of eating disorder patients as the cultivation of neglected souls and psychotherapy as a form of spiritual practice. Rather than focusing on eradicating symptoms or solving problems, the goal of therapy is to bring about meaning, fulfillment, and satisfaction to patients' lives."

This approach is echoed by the authors of an article in a clinical journal, where it was written that, "The role of religious and spiritual influences in human development, functioning, and healing is becoming more widely recognized in the medical and psychological professions" (Richards, 1997). In their article, which reviews numerous studies on spirituality and eating disorders, the authors suggest a variety of activities, some of which are included in the following, expanded list:

RELIGIOUS AND SPIRITUAL ACTIVITIES

- Embrace spiritual concepts like: grace, honesty, and service.

- Read religious or spiritual books, including the scriptures of your chosen religion or "New Age" titles.

- Pray.

- Practice visualization, meditation, and other relaxation techniques that quiet the mind.

- Encourage forgiveness for yourself and others.

- Seek spiritual direction from religious leaders who are positive and uplifting (as opposed to shaming or controlling).

- Get involved in a religious community.

- Do volunteer work or "selfless service."

- Participate in "soulful" activities like inspirational writing, being in nature, musical pursuits, artwork, gardening, etc.

- Keep good company by spending time with others who are interested in spiritual pursuits.

Almost 60% of the bulimics we surveyed mentioned spirituality as being helpful. They usually were deeply inspired and motivated, regardless of their faith. Many specific religions and practices were mentioned, but the underlying message was that recoveries were aided by faith in God as defined by each individual. Some people practiced self-love and love for their "neighbors" with the same spiritual effect and positive consequences.

The main thing that has helped is my faith and trust in God. A lack of security is a problem with eating disorder sufferers and knowing God cares for me gives me comfort and peace. We all need someone to trust, whom we know loves us unconditionally, not for how we look or what we do, just for us as we are.

An eating disorder is just a symptom that something is seriously wrong in our lives. In fact, it is an invitation to grow, emotionally and spiritually. Every crisis is an opportunity.

Today, I am reclaiming my feelings and working very hard to see that I am lovable and valuable. I deserve to live a joyous, fulfilled, serene life. Many times I've gone walking instead of bingeing, and

I've never come home still wanting to binge. Usually I pray while I walk, pouring out all of my burdens, fears, joys, and hopes, knowing that God is hearing me and is delighted in me. I really enjoy this time alone with Him.

Practicing self-love instead of self-pity is important. Having faith and confidence in myself also helps.

Changing Your Mind

People with eating disorders are plagued by negative thinking patterns which maintain their harmful behaviors. This inner chatter goes on constantly, spinning from one topic to another, playing the same destructive "tapes" over and over, and making it impossible to hear anything positive. Bingeing and purging is one way of silencing this relentless critical voice, even if just for a few moments. As Terence Sandbek, author of *The Deadly Diet: Recovering from Anorexia and Bulimia,* writes,

> "Your problems do not stem from your situation, from people or circumstances, but from the way you perceive those people and events. It's your thinking—and not the outside world— that needs to be corrected. So the key to recovery lies in changing your thinking patterns…That's because the Voice—the destructive self-talk that triggers your destructive emotions—just loves to get you so focused on your emotions, your body, and so upset by your environment and the swirl of panic-related symptoms that you can't think straight enough to fight it." (1993)

A few examples of negative thinking patterns are:

- **Seeing everything as black or white.**

Food becomes good or bad; weight gain equals obesity. You always look in the full-length mirror but never like what you see.

- **Magnifying the negatives.**

Filtering out the positives, and letting only the negatives through. Minor problems are seen as catastrophes and comments get blown out of proportion. If you see an increase on the scale, the day is ruined. If someone disagrees with an opinion, you think they hate you.

- **Taking everything personally.**

Thinking that the world revolves around you. If you see a picture in a magazine, you compare whether or not you are thinner. You feel guilty over matters that often have nothing to do with you, or feel that people are judging you or that the world is against you.

- **The "shoulds."**

Having rigid rules about how you and others should act, such as, "Anger should not be expressed," or "I should not eat salad dressing." The "should's" make you think that you control things that might very well be out of your control.

These thought patterns define your existence, in some ways, because what you think is what you experience. If your mind is focused on how bad your life is, then life is bad for you. If you are focused on being ashamed of being bulimic, then shame is your reality. On the other hand, if you make a conscious effort to fight these habitual patterns, you can change how you experience everything. Focusing on what is positive in your life will make you feel more positive. Having compassion for the pain that surely drove you to bulimia will erase the shame. In this way, *what you think has the power to change your life.*

ACTIVITIES FOR CHANGING YOUR MIND

• Listen to what you think and what you say. This might seem like a simplistic idea, but clarity is important in this exercise.

• Practice different, more positive self-talk in your speaking and writing. Try "reframing" thoughts by writing out the negative and countering it with a positive.

• When negative thoughts arise, observe them with non-attachment. You can take note of the ideas, but let them pass without having a mental conversation.

• Make a list of affirmations to say out loud, like "I am a great person." Even if you do not believe these statements 100%, the act of verbalizing will affect you not only emotionally but on a cellular level, as well!

• Practice visualization, meditation, and other relaxation techniques that quiet the mind.

• Accept that you are doing the best you can at the moment. Even bulimia is a way of taking care of yourself when you know of no other. Now, write it a thank-you note and say goodbye.

• Make a list of the ways in which you can take care of yourself. Write yourself a thank you note!

Transforming your thoughts from negative to positive is a powerful tool for change. However, this "mental housecleaning" has the added benefit of making it possible for you to hear your own inner voice more clearly. Although it has probably been quite faint up to now, you do have a quiet voice of wisdom and guidance that comes from the deepest center of your being. It is reassuring, comfortable, wise, fun, confident, and completely trustworthy. The inner voice has only your best interests at heart, which coincidentally is where it resides. It is the voice of your inner self; that pure benevolent force that lies within each of us.

With practice, you will be able to hear this voice more and more clearly. How do you practice? With tenacity and faith, follow the suggestions in this chapter, such as: write in your journal, enhance your self esteem, focus on the positives, express yourself, take time to relax, cultivate relationships and pursue your spirit. It takes work, but the end result will bring you more happiness, better feelings about who you are, and greater contentment with the world. When you take the time to change your mind and open yourself to the inner voice, miracles happen.

I know that I should try a new way of thinking because the old hasn't worked.

Although recovery was the most difficult challenge of my life, I can now experience the beautiful things that I couldn't from the inside of a toilet bowl, like the smell of leaves, butterflies, wild flowers, and how it feels to love myself and others. My mind was clouded with thoughts of eating and throwing up.

I used to feel like I was on automatic pilot. I let my thoughts dictate my life. Now, I dictate what I think!

I like to imagine a paper shredder in my mind where I destroy all the negative thoughts.

Challenging Cultural Influences

We live in a culture that worships thinness. This is not news for anyone, least of all people who suffer from eating disorders. The media is filled with images of thin models who look healthy, happy, successful, smart, and sexy—implying that the key to such a wonderful life is to be thin. Billions of dollars every year are spent by the diet, fashion, and beauty industries to convince women, and increasing numbers of men, to be different from the way they naturally are. The relentless barrage of advertising makes you think that your hair "should" be lighter or bouncier, your teeth "should" be whiter, and you "should" be thinner.

The flip side to our obsession with thinness is a hatred of fat. The media stereotypes fat people as stupid, lacking in willpower, undesirable, and failures. While our society has become more accepting of differences in race, religion, or gender, weight prejudice is still rampant. Bombarded with concepts of thin = good and fat = bad images, it is no wonder that you are terrified of gaining weight and wish to be thinner.

Also, even though we've made strides in the area of women's rights, we still live in a culture that is male oriented. Women are generally lower paid than men, rarely reach high political or corporate positions, are victims of harassment and violence, and are inescapably seen as sexual objects. Bulimia helps women cope with the fear and lack of fulfillment that comes from being devalued and treated as sexual objects or second-class citizens.

What's more, masculine traits such as competitiveness, independence, and aggression are encouraged, while feminine characteristics like being nurturing, interdependent, and cooperative are less valued. An eating disorder can be a way to escape the confusion of what it means to be a woman in a such a male-oriented environment. Men who develop bulimia—whether heterosexual or homosexual—are typically more sensitive than the "average" male, and they, too, use their eating disorder to retreat from such a hostile society.

This theme, which was put forth almost 20 years ago in the classic book, *The Obsession: Reflections on the Tyranny of Slenderness*, by Kim Chernin, is equally true today:

> "A woman obsessed with the size of her body, wishing to make her breasts and thighs and hips and belly smaller and less apparent, may be expressing the fact that she feels uncomfortable being female in this culture." (1981)

Despite decades of advocacy, activists in the women's movement and size-acceptance field, working side by side with eating disorders therapists and educators, have made little progress towards changing our culture's unreasonable standards of beauty and limited gender roles. However, each of us as individuals can choose to rise above cultural obsession and oppression; your recovery mandates that you do so.

TEN WAYS TO CHALLENGE CULTURAL INFLUENCES

- Dieting is a form of oppression; do not diet!
- Notice how television stereotypes people according to weight, and turn off those kinds of shows.

- Tear out and discard magazine photos of skinny women. How many pictures of women are left?

- Write angry letters to advertisers and manufacturers that promote values of thinness; and applaud those that use plus-size models.

- Respect people without regard to their size.

- Don't tolerate negative comments that others make about weight.

- Get involved with, or financially support, organizations that promote size acceptance or eating disorders prevention.

- Don't buy "women's" magazines that promote weight-loss.

- Talk back to the television by verbally denouncing demeaning images.

- Embrace your individuality; assert your own, unique identity.

I had to accept myself and not feel the compelling urge to be "perfect" as reflected by my old need to be "perfectly" slender. I had to acknowledge that with my genes I'd never look like a model; and, that that was okay.

Nobody told me that when girls hit puberty, they put on weight in preparation for childbirth. I thought that I was the only one! When dieting didn't work, I turned to bulimia and was caught for thirteen years. I am now fighting to get my "natural" body back and love it, no matter what its size or shape!

Last year, I made a resolution that I would say something whenever one of my friends mentioned that they felt too fat or wanted to lose weight. It has been hard to be so honest, but when they hear what I have been through, they are a little more accepting of themselves. Even I can be a teacher!

CHAPTER 6

Healthy Eating and Healthy Weight

At some point in your recovery, you will need a plan for eating without fear. When you face the daily decisions about what and how much to eat, knowing the truth about healthy eating and healthy weight will help. So, before discussing meal planning and how to get past food fears, let's review some facts that were mentioned earlier in this book:

FACTS ABOUT HEALTHY EATING & WEIGHT

- Bulimia is not just about food.
- Bodies come in all shapes and sizes; your body type is mostly determined by family genes.
- Everyone has a genetically determined weight range which is naturally best for them—their set point.
- Fat people, on the average, do not eat more than those who are thin.
- Bulimics binge to satisfy emotional hungers not physical ones.

- A healthy, well-balanced diet includes complex carbohydrates, protein, fat, vitamins, and minerals.

- Everyone's body is different, and deciding what and how much you eat will ultimately be up to you.

Dieting and Set Point

Let's acknowledge a crucial fact regarding dieting and weight loss—DIETING DOES NOT WORK. At any given moment, some 20 million Americans are actively dieting, and 95% of them will regain that weight and probably more. Most of those people will blame themselves for this failure, but ultimately it is the premise of losing weight by dieting which is false.

The most basic reason why diets don't work is that the human body has a variety of survival mechanisms designed to maintain its optimal weight. These mechanisms perceive a restriction of food intake as an emergency, like starvation, and make adjustments so that the body holds on to precious pounds instead of letting them go. Let me explain.

Everyone's body has a particular weight range of between about five to ten pounds at which our bodies are the healthiest and work most efficiently. This "set point" or "set point range" can be somewhat influenced by diet, heredity, age, health, and activity level; but generally speaking, *each of us has a natural weight our bodies want to be.* In fact, our body fights to maintain this optimal weight.

Too little food is interpreted as starvation, causing our metabolism to decrease and our body to slow down to preserve calories. On the flip side, a larger amount of food is a signal to speed up the metabolism to compensate for calories that are not needed. In this way, our bodies are working to keep us at a healthy, natural weight. This might be higher or lower than you think it should be, but it is the one your body wants to maintain. So long as you are not starving or stuffing yourself, you can eat a variety of foods—more on some days and less on others—and stay a stable size. Again, this size is not yours to determine, it is only yours to accept and ultimately love.

Another balancing system of the body handles water. Rapid water loss accounts for almost all of the weight decrease during the early stages of a restrictive diet. When the body is deprived of blood sugar via restricted carbohydrate consumption, the liver will first break down its own stored sugar (glycogen), and then will convert amino acids from muscle protein into sugar. Both the glycogen and amino acid molecules are surrounded by water, which is then released from the cells, passes to the kidneys, and is excreted as urine. For this reason, dieters can initially lose several pounds of water weight quickly. However, the kidneys adapt to this water loss by retaining sodium and consequently water. It is this adaptation that many dieters experience as a weight "plateau."

This water-retaining principle combined with a decreased metabolism can cause a weight rebound when you begin to eat normally and your body perceives that it is no longer in danger. Be aware of this! Your body has to go through a period of adjustment to a new way of life, and balancing water and metabolism are crucial. You might experience particularly loud hunger signals or be unsure exactly what or when to eat. This is natural. Follow the meal plan that you have outlined with a nutritionist or dietician and trust your body to take care of you.

Body weight is actually not indicative of having a healthy body. *Research has proven that thinner is not healthier.* In fact, among individuals who are generally fit, those who weigh above the "ideal" standards on weight charts have a significantly lower mortality rate than those who weigh below the "ideal" (Gaesser, 1996). The idea that a large body can be healthy may be a difficult truth to swallow given how brainwashed we have been by the diet and fashion industries, nonsensical insurance company standards, and our misguided prejudice against fat. Having an eating disorder, over-exercising or drastically cutting fats might result in a temporarily lower weight, but will not make you feel better or be healthier physically.

The best way to reach and maintain your set point is through moderate, regular exercise combined with a permanent healthy diet. See below. But restrictive dieting, purging, or any other method of trying to attain a weight that is significantly lower than this set point range will not work. Instead, you will create physical hunger, depression, anger, feelings of deprivation, weakness, loss of focus, and a preoccupation with food—and probable weight gain.

Getting Past Food Fears

Individuals with bulimia usually have strong beliefs and follow self-imposed rules about eating. Straying too far from these patterns is frightening. They label foods "good" or "bad" based on how they think their weight will be affected by eating them. When they eat "bad" foods, they feel like they've broken the rules and are out of control. That often triggers binge eating with the expectation that purging will make everything "good" again. Obviously, it doesn't. In fact, foods are neither "good" nor "bad." Some are more nutritious than others, but that doesn't embody them with inherent value. Eating dessert does not make you a bad person, nor must it lead to bingeing.

You will want to identify some "safe" foods at first. Make a list so you know what you will permit yourself to have without guilt. This establishes a "can-have" rather than a "can't-have" mentality. Gradually, when you are ready, be willing to take some risks and expand that list. Every new food will bring up thoughts and emotions, but you will be able to handle them if you go at your own pace. The negative associations that you attach to foods *can* be recognized and eliminated, especially if they are tackled head on in a systematic and determined manner. Use your journal. Use support people. Do not belittle this challenge! For all the insight into the "whys" of your bulimia, the fact remains that you want to be able to eat without fear. Food is not the enemy.

In many cases, food fears are perpetuated by false beliefs about food and weight. For instance, the idea that eating anything with sugar will cause you to gain weight is not true. Equally false are the beliefs that you should eliminate all fat from your menu or that eating only fruits and vegetables is a healthy vegetarian diet. While these distortions might help preserve a sense of safety and identity, they stand in the way of recovery and must be challenged. Increase the variety and amount of food you eat, with growing confidence.

For some binge eaters, certain foods—especially chocolate— have an addictive effect. Like an alcoholic, these individuals have a psychological dependence and know that by eating their addictive substance, they are apt to lose control. Many of those individuals use the "abstinence" approach to those particular foods.

However, they still must discover new foods to eat because their previous menu was so single-minded.

One method for introducing new foods is to choose one "forbidden" food. Just go for it, even one bite! Concentrate on its texture and flavor. Be persistent about pushing away troublesome thoughts by focusing on the feeling of chewing or the food going down your throat. Remind yourself continually that food is filled with love and you deserve it. When you finish eating, set a timer for ten minutes and allow yourself to have all of the usual habitual thoughts, like "I won't be able to keep this food in; I want to vomit," but don't do it! When the timer goes off, firmly say out loud, "It's only food! Who cares?" Then force yourself to do something else. Perhaps write in your journal, call a friend, or go to a park. Get on with your life.

Be patient with yourself. It takes time to change long-term behaviors and reactions. But it is possible and you can do it. Here are a few ideas to help you get past food fears:

SUGGESTIONS FOR GETTING PAST FOOD FEARS

- Eat for health instead of dieting.
- Affirm that you deserve to eat the best, and that there is plenty.
- If you have setback binges, learn from them.
- Experiment with (even a taste of) different foods and cuisines. A little risk-taking can result in feelings of competence and mastery.
- Try "gentle eating" and appreciating what you eat, instead of gobbling down your meals in a mindless trance.

- To introduce a previously forbidden food, try exchanging it for one of your "safe" foods.

- Perhaps try a new food every week, or promise yourself one delicious dessert every day, week, or month.

- Allow someone else to cook and serve a meal for you.

- Grocery shop with friends to see what foods they like. Talk about your concerns.

- Rely on your support team for reassurance, such as by using an "eating buddy" to sit with you during meals.

- Cook with reverence or serve with style! Does this sound like an advertisement? I'm trying to sell you on eating and enjoying it!

Meal Planning

Many individuals in recovery find it helpful to have a structured approach to their meals. Work with a nutritionist or dietitian who is familiar with eating disorders and its treatment. You want an individualized, balanced eating plan just for you. A professional can give you nutritional information and emotional support, but if professional help is not available or not your choice, you can create your own. Write out which foods you are going to eat, in what proportion, and at what time. Start with foods with which you feel safe, then slowly introduce new foods as you gain confidence. Make an effort to stick to this plan, returning to it even if you stray for a meal.

There's nothing wrong with eating at set intervals while you learn to recognize and respond to physical hunger. Some experts recommend eating three, balanced meals and two or three between-meal snacks daily. There's also nothing wrong with simply eating when you are hungry, once you learn to differentiate between physical and emotional hunger. Some people are comfortable with six small meals, or eating every couple of hours. If sticking to a schedule frees your mind from worries about food, great! If you want more freedom, be flexible. Do what works for you.

A healthy, well-balanced diet includes complex carbohydrates, protein, fat, vitamins, and minerals. Unless a nutritionist or dietitian has given you a meal plan with a specific number of calories, I do not recommend counting calories. Instead, follow your physical hunger signs and use these suggested daily, dietary guidelines, which are based on the recommendations of the US Department of Agriculture:

RECOMMENDED DAILY BALANCED DIET

- 3-5 servings of vegetables. One serving is about a half cup of raw vegetables, a cup of leafy vegetables, or three-quarters of a cup of juice.

- 2-4 servings of fruit. An apple or orange would be about one serving, as would a half grapefruit or three-quarters of a cup of juice.

- 2-3 servings of foods rich in protein, like dairy products, meat, fish, poultry, tofu, or legumes. A cup of milk, a couple of eggs, or 3-4 tablespoons of peanut butter equal one serving.

• 6-11 servings of grains, including: bread, cereal, rice, or pasta. One serving is a slice of bread, ounce of cereal, 2-3 crackers, or half cup of cooked rice or pasta.

• Fatty foods, like mayonnaise, butter, margarine, salad dressing, chocolate, and desserts should not be avoided, but should be eaten more sparingly. Aim for having about 20-30% fat calories in your diet, but don't be rigid about counting calories.

• Drink about 8-10 cups of water.

Special Situations

Eating at restaurants and going to parties can be particularly stressful for individuals with eating disorders. Often, they are reluctant to eat in public and fearful of eating too much. Since many restaurants serve portions that are too large for anyone, you need to be assertive about choosing how much to eat. There are no rules that say you must eat everything that is served to you. If you get anxious in these situations, use a relaxation technique to help get you through the meal, or talk about your fears with supportive companions. If you are served more food than you want, separate what seems to be an appropriate amount on your plate and only eat that much. Another option is to order from the appetizer menu, or share a meal with a friend. If you are uncomfortable about something that is served, you are under no obligation to eat it. Don't panic; relax.

You can't expect to immediately feel at ease eating out; but part of recovery involves getting comfortable with the social aspect of eating. Challenge yourself by making and accepting invitations. Eventually, you might come to enjoy going out for meals with friends.

I told myself that there will always be cheesecake or chocolate, bread, whatever! If I don't eat it now it won't be gone forever.

I remember being terrified about going to restaurants when I had bulimia, but now I love eating out and hosting dinner parties.

I allow myself anything I want, but in moderation. I have cake and ice cream, bread and butter, even cream in my coffee. The serving size is appropriate to my needs at the time. Being able to allow myself anything to eat has taken away the guilt, where before one bite of a "forbidden food" would lead to a binge; I eat it, enjoy it, and keep it down.

There are no forbidden foods for me. Certain foods don't have the power that I once gave them.

I try to eat several times a day in small portions. The foods that I eat now leave me feeling satisfied, and I have no desire to binge.

Allowing myself all foods, in small quantities, has helped me, although I must remind myself I "deserve" cakes, cookies, etc. Cutting out all sugars set me up to binge, which reinforced that I was "bad" and couldn't control myself. I pretended not to eat sugar and carbohydrates, only to binge on them in private. I now eat sweets in small amounts in front of everyone, not trying to be "perfect" in my diet.

Health is my priority, not thinness.

CHAPTER 7

Things to Do
Instead of Bingeing

Even though an eating disorder causes tremendous pain and suffering, giving it up is difficult. Anyone who has gone through it will agree. You will undoubtedly face challenges and even hardships along the way, but no matter how hard it seems, the rewards are there: time for friends, money for fun, energy to feel a full range of emotions, clarity to know your inner truth, more love!

Take a moment to think about why you want to stop your bulimia. As a matter of fact, take a piece of paper and draw a vertical line down the middle. On the left side of the line, write "Bulimia" and all of your reasons for wanting to keep it. On the right, list your reasons for wanting to give it up. Are you willing to trade? Maybe? On a scale of one to ten, how willing are you? Enough to start now, I hope.

At the same time, understand that you can't give up something if you don't have something else to put in its place. What will you do instead of bulimia? This is important to think about because you need to be ready. Make some connections with other people who can support you. Get the books ready that you will read, the candles for your hot baths, new hiking shoes if nature is to be your teacher. Make your plan and gather the necessary "tools" that you will need to put something in place of your former rituals and habits.

Below are some suggestions for "things to do" which have helped thousand of others, and they can help you, too. There are three lists, each with a different purpose. When you are tempted to binge, pick one idea from the "Immediate" list below, and do it! Use the "Short-term" list afterwards for planning how not to binge in the future, and the "Long-term" list for larger, lifestyle changes. Personalize these lists in any way, at any time, by adding your own ideas. After all, it's *your* recovery.

If you are committed to recovery, stopping yourself from bingeing and purging is imperative. Regardless of how you eventually address the underlying issues, you still must make a stand now. Make a copy of the "Immediate" list and put it on your refrigerator. When you are tempted to binge, select an item from the list instead. Also, there are many more ideas like these in the "Three-Week Program to Stop Bingeing" in Chapter Nine.

IMMEDIATE THINGS TO DO INSTEAD OF BINGEING

• Postpone the binge for 15 minutes. Set your timer. That should give you enough time to choose another strategy.

• Brush your teeth; take a shower or bath.

• Soak binge food in water.

• Leave the environment that's tempting you to binge. Go to a park, library, or other "safe" place.

• Call a supportive friend either just to talk or to

address your problem. Cultivate more friends who are sensitive, compassionate, and capable of up-lifting you. Someone who has overcoming an eating disorder will be especially empathic.

• In panic situations, relax with deep breathing. Take a deep breath for the count of ten, hold it for that long, exhale. Repeat this a few times, then think through your anxiety. What am I feeling? Can I handle what's going on? Am I safe?

• Get your mind on something else. Chew gum. Turn on the radio or television. Distract yourself from the cravings long enough to settle down.

• Let out your emotions in an aggressive way. Punch a boxing bag or scream into a pillow. Wrestle with a safe support person. Beat your bed with a tennis racket or baseball bat. Loud crying can be a great release.

• Take part in physical activity. Go for a walk, jog, swim, or bike ride. Hit golf balls or play tennis.

• Stop yourself and identify the real hunger. Where is it coming from? Throat? Stomach? Heart? Write down your most spontaneous answers. These identify the source of your legitimate wants and needs.

• Write in your journal or tape record thoughts. Be intimate and honest. Look back at earlier entries to discover patterns and see progress. Address questions like, "What's the payoff to this binge?"

• List the foods you are fantasizing about, seal the paper in an envelope, and throw it away.

• Create and use panic cards with step-by-step instructions on what to do in difficult situations. Each card would include one strategy, like "Work in the garden: 1. Go to the nursery and buy seeds, starter plants, or soil amendment. 2. Return home and do planting. 3. Offer your gratitude and blessings to the garden. 4. Show off your work to a friend or neighbor." Come up with a deck of panic cards of your own, including some of the ideas from Chapter Five.

• For incentive, every day you don't binge or purge, mark your calendar with a big star or put money in a jar. When you reach certain goals—whether they're shorter or longer term—give yourself rewards.

• If you can, stop yourself in the middle of a binge. This may seem impossible, but those who have done it say it is a very powerful accomplishment. Try to breathe peace into your uncomfortably full body. Do whatever it takes to stop yourself from eating more or purging. Afterward, process your feelings in your journal or with a support person.

SHORT-TERM PLANNING FOR NOT BINGEING

• Make your own list of "Immediate" things to do instead of bingeing. As you discover which activities are successful, repeat them and add options of a similar vein.

• Incorporate relaxation techniques into your daily routine. Take a yoga class, meditate for 20 minutes every morning and night, or simply take "Quiet Time" to be away from others and alone with your thoughts.

• Give yourself permission to eat what you crave, but do it with a capable support person who understands your goal is to increase self-awareness, not to binge. Spend time talking about your feelings or writing them down. Do not purge.

• Investigate your childhood. Everyone has deep issues related to their family and the environment in which they were raised. Our relationships with friends and teachers, the way we viewed media and culture, and so much more are also part of who we are today. Look through photo albums and memorabilia, ask questions of your parents, share notes with friends and siblings, and devote time to reflect. Uncover any causes for your bulimia that you can.

• Write a letter to a family member about your bulimia; however, *you do not have to send the letter.* Have the courage to say who you are and what you need. Write a series of letters to that person over an extended period of time. Be honest, assertive, and candid.

• Call or visit a "long lost" childhood friend whom

you have thought about over the years but haven't seen. Track them down. Catch up on each other's life. They will not judge you for your bulimia; they have their own unique stories to tell.

• Eat "normally" for one day using the guidelines in Chapter Six, and observe what you eat and how that feels. Could you get used to eating that way?

• Plan ahead and attend a cultural event, like a concert, art exhibit, stage play, or museum. Prior to going, study up on the subject. For example, if you are going to hear a symphony, listen to it beforehand and read up on the composer. These kinds of personally enriching activities can take the place of bingeing.

• Make lists about your life: likes and dislikes, goals, priorities, accomplishments, things-to-do, people to call, etc. Lists are good for organizing your thoughts instead of letting them spin.

• Practice saying "No." Be assertive and express your needs, small or large. Set your own limits and boundaries. This may feel risky at first, but it gets easier as you get stronger. Always remember, you have a fundamental human right to your own opinions and decisions.

• Take a vacation. Get away from your usual routine, and decide not to binge and purge while away. Be a "new" you while you are gone, and think about ways to continue with that attitude when you return home. You may discover it worthwhile to make changes to your regular environment.

• Try visual imagery, which can help you to later act out a situation in a positive way. Picture yourself doing something before you do it. For example, before dinner, mentally see yourself walking into the kitchen, preparing a healthy meal, eating it in a pleasant setting, and cleaning up afterward. Imagine that scenario as purely enjoyable. Then replicate it in reality.

• Begin to smile at others. Consider hugging! Remember that most people are a bit shy themselves. Something as small as a nod of the head or tip of a hat can connect you in a wonderful way.

LONG-TERM THINGS TO DO TO END BULIMIA

• Get involved in volunteer work. Offer to help out at a retirement center, school, environmental agency, animal shelter, or political office. By giving freely, your own goodness will radiate back to you.

• Practice love by taking care of pets. A dog or cat will provide unconditional acceptance, affection, and companionship. Staring at fish can be relaxing. People have all kinds of pets for all kinds of reasons.

• Learn something new: a foreign language, CPR, a musical instrument, an art medium, mechanics or electronics, or computer programs. Try out classes which emphasize self-reliance, assertiveness, or improved body image.

• Think about how to make more money instead of obsessing about food, and then follow through on your scheme. This can be a hobby, investment plan, or a new career.

• Read! Go to the library or local bookstore. Always have a book to read for pleasure (novel, biography, history, etc.).

• Use positive language. Try saying out loud that you are a nice person and deserve to live happily. Talk into a tape recorder. Repeat affirmations.

• Try not to be so perfect. Bulimics are often tidy about everything except their own inner peace. Concentrate on the needs of your inner self. Don't be so finicky about housework or study so much. Stop wearing makeup to see how that feels.

• Begin to record your dreams on paper. Watch for patterns and subtle meanings. If it interests you, get a book on dream analysis.

• Experiment with your own interests!

CHAPTER 8

Advice for Loved Ones

A few words from Leigh:

Lindsey and I fell in love at first sight. Shortly after we acknowledged our love, she told me she had a "horrible" secret. I was a bit relieved when it turned out to be "only" an eating disorder. But when she fully described the scope of her bingeing and vomiting, I realized that I had underestimated its seriousness. Actually, at that time, the word "bulimia" was not even commonly used, and no one realized how widespread it was.

I quickly discovered that there was no instantaneous cure for Lindsey's bulimia, and we both feared that unless she gave it up, our relationship was jeopardized. For nine years, it had monopolized her time and attention, and prevented her from appreciating the goodness within herself that I recognized so immediately. Although I was ignorant about eating disorders, I responded with compassion and my pledge to help with her recovery. She allowed me to be supportive.

Lindsey's battle with bulimia was our primary focus for many months as she worked to put it behind her. During that time, I had to continually remind myself that becoming free was up to her. I could make suggestions, be a sounding board, or even take punches with the boxing gloves, but I was not the one who had to do the work. I could not "fix" her. Of course, I was not merely an unaffected bystander—our union was predicated on her recovery. Also, her struggles forced me to examine my own values on such subjects as family relationships, weightism, stereotypes in the media, feminism, and healthy eating. Still, I never lost sight of the fact that she was the one in crisis.

Sometimes people who have heard her story give me more credit than is due. I merely provided support and ideas—the same kinds of suggestions that fill this book. I didn't have difficulties with food or self esteem, so I never experienced firsthand the pain or the courage that Lindsey encountered. Instead, I reaped the benefits of her dedication to recovery. Consequently, our love has flourished for more than twenty years, and I stumbled onto my life's work. I never expected that I would write and publish books on eating disorders for a career, or that I would interact with thousands of people concerned with food problems. I have been fortunate to be able to help many of them and their loved ones, and am confident that the advice we offer in this chapter can be helpful to you.

GENERAL SUGGESTIONS

- Remember that she (or he) has the food problem, and it is up to them to do the work.

- Make a pact of complete honesty.

- Be patient, sympathetic, non-judgmental, and a good listener. Let her know that you care and have her best interests at heart.

• Accept that recovery is a process and does not happen quickly. Help her to be patient, as well.

• Do not be controlling of her life; you are limited in what you can do to help. You may need to learn about letting go.

• When her behavior affects you, express yourself without placing guilt or blame upon her. Try not to take her actions personally. Use "I" messages, explaining your feelings and concerns. You may need to disengage from her to take care of yourself.

• Have compassion. Your loved one may be overwhelmed as she gets in touch with the painful issues underlying the behavior. She will need your love and support at these times more than ever.

• Always remind yourself that your loved one uses bulimia as a substitute for confronting painful feelings or experiences. Ask what, if anything, you can do to help. Encourage her to find healthier ways to deal with her pain.

• Do not try to guess what she wants. Encourage her to express her needs. If you have questions, ask.

• Encourage her to enter professional therapy, keeping in mind that no single approach to recovery works for everyone. Be available for joint counseling. Be flexible and open in supporting her to do whatever approaches she chooses. For example, you may know someone who goes to a particular therapist, but your loved one might relate better to another.

- Recognize that she needs to learn to make her own decisions, and that the direction of her recovery is her responsibility. Don't constantly check up on her unless she asks that of you.

FOOD AND EATING

- Remember that food is not the problem, and bulimia is a symptom. Look past the immediate situation to the deeper issues.

- Allow her to establish reasonable rules and goals about food and eating, but assert your rights as well. Only make rules that can be enforced; work within a framework that will result in successes rather than failures.

- Make it clear that she is responsible for the consequences of her bulimic behavior. For example, if she binges on the family's food, she should replace it using her own money. If she vomits, she should clean the bathroom. If she steals, she must make amends.

- If she binges, she should face it afterwards by talking about why it happened, writing in a journal, or exploring options for how to avoid bingeing the next time she is in a similar situation.

- Do not allow meals to be a battleground. Avoid turning her eating into a power struggle. Mealtime conversations should not revolve around her bulimia.

• Encourage the bulimic to develop a safe and healthy meal plan on her own or with a nutritionist or dietician. Support her every small step.

• Don't talk about her appearance. You may think you are offering compliments, but those can be interpreted in different ways. For example, if you tell her she looks "pretty" she can take that to mean that she usually looks ugly. Saying she looks thin only puts a destructive overemphasis on weight.

• Plan activities that do not revolve around food. Take walks together, visit museums, go to the movies, play sports. If she is uncomfortable about eating, then do something besides going to restaurants for entertainment.

• Do not make food decisions for the bulimic. Those are up to her. Be supportive of her choices. For example, if she is not eating desserts and you are, don't expect her to prepare them or purchase them for you. Do that on your own.

FOCUS ON YOU

• Consider getting professional help for yourself. Having a child or other loved one with an eating disorder is one of the most stressful situations imaginable. Take care of yourself, and you will be a better support to those around you.

• Be open to the possibility that you are somehow contributing to her problem, and that you

might need to challenge some of your own behaviors and beliefs.

• Learn about eating disorders and related issues,
such as: societal pressures on women, the exploi-
tation of thinness, weight prejudice, set point, family dynamics, and self esteem.

• Read the book, *Surviving an Eating Disorder:
Strategies for Family and Friends* by Michele Siegel,
Judith Brisman, and Margot Weinshel. This and
many other helpful titles are available from the
Eating Disorders Resource Catalogue (see last
page).

On our survey of recovered and recovering bulimics we asked,
"What can family and friends do to help?" The responses provide
more excellent guidelines:

*The best way for loved ones to help me is just love me and be there
when I need them.*

*Be honest and supportive of the person finding a cure, without
supporting the behavior.*

*Look at how you feel about food or if you contribute to your loved
one's bulimia.*

*I'm firmly convinced that loved ones first need to admit that this is
a serious problem and that it takes a great deal of sometimes un-
pleasant work for the bulimic to get better.*

Communication is very important! The person who is bulimic needs to be able to freely discuss any feelings and concerns that she might have—without feeling threatened.

Loved ones can encourage, love, support, and actively listen. I found that some people listen for about 60 seconds and then interject their opinions and prejudices instead of openly listening and really hearing what is said.

They can de-emphasize food and support the concept that a woman is beautiful even if she weighs more than a model. They have to realize that models are not the standard of beauty.

Be there for me! Isolation and loneliness just worsen the problem. Help me to build self esteem and self worth. Notice the good things and comment on them instead of harping on the bad.

Loved ones need to help bulimics assert themselves. I needed reassurance that it was okay to say "No" to people.

Recognize that the bulimic's perfectionism and conscientiousness hide a deep sense of inferiority and self-doubt. Draw her out of her "authoritarian cocoon." Speak your mind!

Try to learn about the disorder, especially the underlying issues and causes.

Encourage the bulimic to go into therapy.

Be patient and do not expect "instant" results.

Offer to pay for therapy!

My loved ones can best help by showing their love for me both in words and actions. I especially need to know they love me in spite of my bingeing and purging. Please don't lecture me or tell me I'm sick. I know loving me isn't easy, but please try! I need your love! I need to be accepted and smiled at.

Never make a big deal about food, which is not the main issue anyway. The sooner the family realizes this, the sooner they can help the bulimic, herself, realize it as truth.

CHAPTER 9

A Three-Week Program
to Stop Bingeing

The purpose of this section is to give someone with bulimia specific goals and tasks to help them stop abusing food. This program is not an instant cure, but rather an experience of what it might feel like to be well. It can also provide insights into the recovery process for other readers who are interested, and is equally appropriate for men or women.

The course requires spending time and effort. Even if you are not ready to do the full program or even one daily routine, you can benefit from trying some of the techniques. We recommend the same things that we talk about in this book—doing things instead of bingeing, journal writing, relaxation, moderate exercise, professional therapy, talking to people, etc.

Skim through the entire chapter first, and the format will become clear to you. On various days, you will practice having fun, being loving, thinking happy thoughts, and getting to know yourself better. If you use this plan faithfully, you will have developed some skills and confidence to help you stop your bulimia for good. At the very least, your bingeing will decrease during the three-week course; and even if you do binge, you will not have failed. You will learn new ways to understand why you had a setback and will be given guidelines to prevent the next binge. We are providing a framework for your continued recovery. We attempt to be inspiring, but clearly you are the one who will do the work.

Obviously, you have a life apart from bulimia, but can still do this program if you also have a job, go to school, or have other important responsibilities. Hopefully, time for the assignments will come from time *not* spent planning and executing binges. Feel free to rearrange the order of days to accommodate your usual, busy routine.

Let us remind you again that your bulimia has served you in many ways, most notably to protect you from painful feelings. Experiencing past hurts, present shame, or other unfamiliar, un-expressed emotions can be frightening and overwhelming. More-over, if you are not used to having feelings or even differentiating one from another, you may be tempted to turn to your familiar friend, bulimia, for safety. Can you understand how natural this is? Can you have compassion for yourself given the task ahead?

Our advice is to be aware and prepared. Have someone or something to support you—a therapist, friend or relative, pet, eating disorders support group either on-line or in person, cas-sette tapes of your own soothing voice or special music, hotline or local treatment phone number in case of emergency, or other books. Come up with your own list and use it.

In this fifth edition of *Bulimia: A Guide to Recovery* we have expanded the "Program to Stop Bingeing" from two to three weeks because readers wanted more. Following are excerpts from a few of the letters we've received from people who tried the original, two-week program. We feel blessed knowing that individuals like yourself, who want to recover from bulimia, will be using this course. We hope that it can help you. Give it a try!

I am seventeen years old and am on Day 13 of your two-week program. How can I begin to thank you? It's weird, at first I didn't want to do the program or even read the book. I felt like I didn't have a problem. Now I can recognize negative thoughts and say "NO! I will not give in to this excuse of a disease! Bulimia is something I have control over and I will not let it win! Thank you for caring, you are true angels.

I have been in and out of treatment and am trying to recover. Whenever I find myself relapsing, I use your two-week program to get myself back on the right track.

Just a note to say thank you. You were both a great inspiration to me when I made the decision to begin recovery from bulimia. Your book has been a blessing. I have just completed the last chapter and it has been two weeks and I can honestly say things are looking a lot brighter. I feel more in touch with myself and who I truly am. I have learned how to humble myself and ask for support when I need it.

I have just completed the two-week program and am going through it for the second time starting today.

I found your book to be very useful, especially the two-week recovery program. It helped me to set aside time for myself each day. I have worked through it slowly, actually taking three months. Your book has helped me so much I carry it and my notebook with me just about all the time. I feel more secure with it and know some day I can leave it on a shelf and refer to it from time to time. For now, though, I keep it with me and do homework assignments I hadn't gotten to yet. I wanted you to know how your book has helped me and given me a structured way to focus on my needs. Thank you so much.

🎗 *DAY 1* 🎗

My life is better without bulimia!

Yes! You are making a commitment to end your bulimia and you'll be happy that you did! Since this is your first day, we will have orientation. In the future, the instructions will not include as many details. If Day 1 begins in the afternoon, do everything anyway. Tomorrow, though, you will need to start Day 2 at the beginning of the day. Be prepared to spend some money for materials and field trips. These costs are generally low, and by the end of the course you will have saved money that you probably would have spent on food. Also, Days 9 and 10 may require planning in advance or rescheduling.

Important note: This program offers you the experience of freedom from bulimia. This is *not* a test. There are no right or wrong ways to do it. Stick to it faithfully or choose any of these activities and give them a try.

YOUR NOTEBOOK

Today, buy a three-ring notebook, five dividers, and paper specifically for this course. Keep it and this book next to your bed, and as soon as you get up in the morning, turn to the appropriate page and get started. If you are using a computer, put printouts into your notebook.

Every day you will have written assignments, places to go, or exercises to do. These can be accomplished at any time, before or after meals, instead of bingeing, whenever you can. We strongly suggest that you do all of the assignments, but there may be days when you simply cannot. Do each day's work that day, and if necessary, catch up later.

Arrange your notebook with five dividers labeled:

- Journal
- Things to Do Instead of Bingeing
- Successes & Lessons
- Written Homework
- Other

Today, we will explain about each section:

- Journal

This program has specific journal writing assignments, but you should also feel free to use this space whenever you have something to say. A journal is a sacred, safe place for you to write your innermost thoughts and feelings. It will support you by being a good "listener" and by showing you the patterns and progress of your journey. Always copy the Thought for the Day into it. If you already use a journal, still use this section of your notebook for the program.

- Today's Things to Do Instead of Bingeing

Every day we will provide a few suggestions for things you can do instead of bingeing. You should also write some of your own ideas. Emphasize techniques that work. Record how successful the various options are for you. One requirement of this course is that you consult this list if you are on the verge of a binge.

- Successes & Lessons

Reward yourself with a sheet in this section when you resist the temptation to binge. You might describe your feelings about not bingeing, what alternatives worked for you, or add words of wisdom that may have inspired or entertained you that day.

What if you do binge? Don't give up! Would you quit school if you received a poor grade on one assignment? No, you would study a little harder next time. *Here is your extra homework if you binge:*

1. Write about the binge. Include answers to some of these questions: What led you to do the binge? What were your thoughts before, during, or after? What did you eat? Did you purge? How? What were you feeling? Did you try to do something instead of bingeing? Why didn't that work? What else could you have done? What will you try to do instead of bingeing next time the cravings are so strong?

2. Attach a photo that reminds you of the binge. Some ideas: cut out a magazine advertisement for junk food and put a big black X over it, write over a diet advertisement with the words "Weight is not important to me, loving myself is!" or add a news clipping that reminds you that you are still better off than some unfortunate people.

3. Spend ten minutes relaxing.

- Written Homework

Use this section for keeping your written assignments.

- Other

This section is for additional writing, clippings, souvenirs, etc.

FIRST THINGS FIRST

Every day, as soon as you can, but definitely before eating, you have a few things to do (in order):

1. Glance through each day's entire plan.
2. Read the Thought for the Day.
3. Do the Morning Warm-up.

THOUGHT FOR THE DAY

My life is better without bulimia!

Keep repeating this thought over and over all day. Say it to yourself when you sit down and when you stand up, when you open doors, while driving or washing your hands, continuously when you eat, etc. Every day you will be given another thought. Say it with conviction and belief, and most of all, repeat it!

THE MORNING WARM-UP

If you have to go to the bathroom, you may. If you have roommates, spouses, kids, or others that require your attention, make them wait. Afford yourself this bit of time.

Today, let's start with a good stretch. It will take about ten minutes. Put on some music, if you wish. Here are some hints for getting the most from stretching:

1. Instead of copying someone else's routine, make up your own as you go along. Unlearn rules about keeping joints straight or repetitions.

2. Don't bounce or try to be flexible. Relax and enjoy feeling your muscles. Touch them with your fingers.

3. Groan, sigh, laugh, and breathe noisily—it's fun and releases tension.

4. Slowly stretch your whole body.

5. If you feel tension in your face, there is tension in your body—relax your face!

6. Don't over stretch. If it starts to hurt, relax, breathe, and don't push yourself to go further than you can. Stretching should feel good!

7. Give yourself about ten minutes. Include your eyes, neck, back, shoulders, chest, arms, fingers, thighs, calves, and feet. Alternate bending and arching your back, twisting one direction and then the other, etc. Also, remember to keep repeating the Thought for the Day: "My life is better without bulimia!"

TODAY'S THINGS TO DO INSTEAD OF BINGEING

If you feel compelled to binge, try any of these activities instead. Keep track of what works in the "Things to Do" section in your notebook.

1. Punch, kick, yell, and go wild! Use inanimate objects, such as beds and pillows, boxing bags, or a hammer and wood. Vent your frustrations and tensions, and loudly express those feelings which you've been swallowing. Look at a clock and go three rounds of two minutes each. Make that pillow feel your anger, beat the #$&!! out of it!

2. Get away, quick! Go to a quiet restful place where food is not easily available, such as a park, beach, museum, church, or library. Bring your notebook and write in your journal.

3. Use the relaxation or meditation techniques described earlier in Chapter Five.

4. Exercise! Be sure to stretch first, and pace yourself—don't overexert. If you have a favorite way of exercising, do that. Otherwise, lightly jog, walk, or take a long bicycle ride. Do not use exercise as a purge, and spend from 20 minutes to an hour or so. Isn't that about how long you might spend on a binge?

5. List three options of your own, and do one of those.

HOMEWORK: DAY 1

1. Write about your bingeing habits of the last weeks, months, or years. Include frequency of binges and purges, and describe in detail your last binge. You will refer to this assignment later during the course, so be sure to leave it in the "Written Homework" section.

2. List the various ways in which your life would be better without the bulimia. Be both general and detailed. For instance, you would have more time and money, but time and money for what? Your health would improve, but in what way? Then put assignment #1 next to assignment #2 and compare. Would you like to trade one for the other?

3. Write a final journal entry before going to sleep tonight. Include what you did today, how you felt, and some reflections on this course. Be sure to write, "My life is better without bulimia!" Life really is better without it.

GOOD NIGHT

If today was hard for you, stick to it, because as the days progress, the program will help you stop bingeing. Even if we haven't met personally, we want you to know that we care about you and completely support your efforts. We encourage you to write us about your experiences, and we will write back! Remember to read Day 2 as soon as you wake up, but rest with the knowledge that you are worthwhile, strong, and are on the right track toward ending your bulimia. Sleep well.

⚜ *DAY 2* ⚜

Look for solutions, not problems

Good morning! We hope you slept well and are excited about continuing this program. Let's get started.

THOUGHT FOR THE DAY

Look for solutions, not problems.

Your mind is a creative force. Whatever it thinks about is what is happening for you at that moment—abundance or scarcity, happiness or worry, self-hate or self-esteem. Notice your belittling thoughts and get rid of them. You are not unworthy, you just think that you are. Changing your thoughts will actually change your experience. Today, look on the bright side; in other words, look for solutions, not problems!

THE MORNING WARM-UP

Take a long, hot shower or bath. By all means, sing at least part of one song out loud. Gently stretch and massage yourself as you bathe. Think about what we've planned for you to do today, what you will write about in your journal, and what will be acceptable for you to eat for breakfast.

SHORT JOURNAL ENTRY

Describe one of the happiest moments of your life. Try to remember why you felt so good about yourself then. We want you to remember that good feeling throughout the day.

TODAY'S THINGS TO DO INSTEAD OF BINGEING

1. Gather your binge food and soak it with water in the sink. Don't concern yourself with the waste; you would have wasted it by purging.

2. Take another shower or bath, repeating everything that you did in the Morning Warm-up.

3. Drink water or eat a carrot.

4. Tell yourself to slow down. Spend 15 to 30 minutes in deep relaxation, meditation, or taking a slow walk in a beautiful place.

5. Review yesterday's options and your own list. Choose something that will work!

HOMEWORK: DAY 2

1. Begin compiling your *support list*. Getting support is one way of looking for solutions.

Make one list of all the people who already know about your bulimia. Make another list of everyone you will tell. This list should include practically everyone who is close to you. You do not have to contact these people yet, so there will be some time to get used to this idea. Now, make a loose order of those you will contact first, second, etc. Next to their names, indicate the probable method of contact that you will use, such as: phone call, letter, in-person, etc.

2. When you begin to let go of the bulimia, you will need other activities, thoughts, and feelings to take its place. Today, begin thinking about something *new* you want to learn. This learning will not have to end at the completion of these three weeks. Some ideas: yoga, a musical instrument, a foreign language or computer program, figure drawing, CPR, skydiving, etc. You will be required to spend some time on this, so it should be a fun activity for you.

3. Go for a long walk in your neighborhood. Weather is no obstacle; a brisk walk in the rain or snow can be invigorating. Bring your notepad to record any ideas that you have during the walk. Stop to smell the roses! Smile and talk to people you see; look them in the eye. Observe everything, even the sky. Do not eat or go into any stores during this walk.

Important note: We often recommend that you "get away" in order to avoid a binge, but when you return home it is important to maintain the feelings that kept you from bingeing. As soon as you return, sit quietly for five minutes and relax. After that, write in your journal. Other choices are to call someone, drink a cup of hot tea, take a shower or bath, or do whatever else works for you. As helpful as it is to get away, it is crucial to maintain your positive feelings and commitment to recovery when you return to your usual environment.

GOOD NIGHT

You might be experiencing some joy and sense of accomplishment. Or, you may be frustrated and anxious. Regardless of how it went, another day has passed. Reaffirm that you will continue this program. You can do it! You are doing it! As you drift off to sleep tonight, remember that moment of happiness we asked you to write about earlier? Put yourself in that situation, feel the warmth and love. Somewhere nearby, we are there too, thinking of you as a wonderful, loving person. Sweet dreams!

🐉 *DAY 3* 🐉

Lighten up!

Today is going to be a fun day. Everyone has a sense of humor, but sometimes life's pressures prevent us from having a good laugh. Today, laugh! It feels great! Rearrange your schedule if necessary to get the most enjoyment out of today's assignments.

THOUGHT FOR THE DAY

Lighten up!
(This has nothing to do with your weight!)

People with bulimia tend to be so serious. They look at their lives through depressed eyes and sour expressions. Remember what it feels like to laugh. Try to have a brighter outlook today, even if somber thoughts are lurking in the background. Force yourself to be more lighthearted and more at ease with the flow of the world around you.

THE MORNING WARM-UP

Bring a watch or clock into the bathroom with you and lock the door. Spend five full minutes looking at your face in the mirror—set a timer. Try not to look away. Make extended eye contact with yourself. Who is that? When is the last time you really looked at your face? Look at all of the colors in your eyes. How long has it been since you've noticed that? When you look at someone else, on what do you base your judgments? What kinds of judgments do you make about yourself? How about making some positive affirmations about yourself instead?

While you're at it, make dopey faces in the mirror. Stretch your face, wiggle your lips, squish your nose, pull on your ears, etc. Grunt, squeak, say "Ho ho ho," "ha ha ha," and "he he he." Laugh out loud, even if it's a phony laugh. Come on, lighten up, really get silly!

Also, since you're in the bathroom, talk out loud to your scale if you have one. Tell it that you resent its influence over you. Have a good heart-to-heart with it and consider saying goodbye! Read today's Homework #4.

TODAY'S THINGS TO DO INSTEAD OF BINGEING

1. Write several affirmations in your journal 15 times each, such as: "I won't binge today," "Lighten up!" or "Every day in every way I'm getting better and better." As long as you are still tempted to binge, keep writing!

2. Write a note to someone on your support list telling them that you are participating in this program. You can send it or not.

3. Go for a walk.

4. Do one of today's assignments. There's a lot to do today.

5. Review what has worked and been suggested before.

HOMEWORK: DAY 3

1. These first two homework assignments can be done at a bookstore, library, or on-line. Research what you will need to help you start your new learning project, which was mentioned in yesterday's homework.

2. Also read through joke books or websites. Laugh out loud right there in the aisle or at your desk. Spend no time in the "diet" or "cooking" sections. If you're really ambitious, also go to a music or video store and buy or rent a comedy recording.

3. Contact someone from your support list to tell some of the new jokes that you read today. This isn't necessarily the time to talk about your bulimia, but that would be okay, too.

4. Stop weighing yourself so often. Since you considered saying goodbye this morning, why not destroy your home scale? A hammer will work just fine, though running over it with a car may be equally satisfying. Don't just throw it away. Destroy it and laugh! You need never be controlled by a number again.

GOOD NIGHT

We hope that this day has been as enjoyable for you as it has been for us. We had a few good giggles from the plan. Did you?

〰️ *DAY 4* 〰️

I can eat without fear!

You may have noticed that we haven't said much about food or eating yet. Today, we will. Whatever the causes of your bulimia—whether they be related to family, society, chemical imbalance, karma, a desire to be thin, or anything else—you still need to eat. Don't wait to understand all your "why's" because that in itself will not stop you from bingeing. Begin to appreciate food for its taste and nourishment, and let go of your negative, obsessive thoughts.

THOUGHT FOR THE DAY

I can eat without fear.

Today, you will be facing food choices, preparation and eating, and you will need to be more brave than you've been since your food obsessions started. Truly believing that you can eat without fear day in and day out may take time, but by repeating this affirmation, you are setting a goal and encouraging it to happen. Every time will make you stronger.

THE MORNING WARM-UP

Do a short, five minute stretch. Reread the guidelines from Day 1 if necessary.

MORNING JOURNAL ENTRY

Plan today's menu. Include as many meals as you'd like (breakfast, lunch, dinner, snacks, dessert), but be specific—you will go shopping for groceries later. Your meals today should be balanced, tasty, and nonthreatening. Stick to this menu faithfully. It will give you the experience of using a meal plan.

TODAY'S THINGS TO DO INSTEAD OF BINGEING

1. Buy a plant or new pet, such as a goldfish.

2. Call someone from your support list.

3. Work on your new study project or today's assignments.

4. Ask yourself: What's the payoff to bingeing? How does that compare with the satisfaction of not bingeing? Make a list.

5. Remember a time when you did something brave. Prepare yourself for today's homework by recalling how that felt.

6. As always, review the other days' options.

HOMEWORK: DAY 4

1. Take a name or two from the support list you compiled on Day 2. Reach out to them. If you're nervous, write out some of what you will say first. Include questions that you want to ask, and specific things that you want them to do for you. *It is vital to have a support person to call when you are craving a binge.*

2. Go grocery shopping. Make a detailed list and buy only the food you need for the menu that you have prepared. Do not buy anything that is not on your list. Stick to your menu. You can do it!

3. Bring paper or a notepad to the grocery. In it, write down the name and price of every item of food that you would eat on a binge. Total your savings by not bingeing. Then, either burn the list, tear it up, or eat it (not really)!

4. Have a special meal today. Eat by candlelight and soft music, use good china, prepare a beautiful place setting. Practice gentle, mindful eating. Put your utensil down between bites, taste your food, savor each morsel.

5. If you have not done so already, start making arrangements for at least one session of professional therapy. Reread the answers to "How should I choose a therapist?" in Chapter One. At the least, make a list of potential therapists from referrals or the

phone book. If you are willing, make a few calls and schedule an appointment—the sooner the better.

GOOD NIGHT

Many people say that food is not the issue for bulimics. While we agree with this in principal, we still emphasize that reformed eating habits are crucial for recovery. The binge-purge behavior was learned, now it must be unlearned. You can eat without fear. Let your friends help you and believe in yourself. Stick to this program! Even if we've never met you, we care about you, we really do.

🦋 DAY 5 🦋

Think lovely thoughts!

The suggestions that we make day-to-day require you to work all day, not just for a few moments while you read the page or do an assignment. The effort that you put into them determines how much they affect you. Think about your recovery activities and goals as you eat, rest, bathe, walk, talk, etc. Changing how you think is a deliberate, ever-deepening practice which will affect your life on many other levels.

THOUGHT FOR THE DAY

Think lovely thoughts.

See positives in everyone and everything. If you begin to have a negative thought, stop and replace it with a positive one. Consciously and actively practice feelings of love, approval, and confidence.

THE MORNING WARM-UP

See yourself a little differently. Spend about 20 minutes doing this relaxation exercise: In a quiet place, lie on your back, eyes closed. You will tense and then relax every part of your body. Start with your toes and feet, flexing them, holding the tension, and then releasing, allowing that area to gently relax. Follow this procedure up your calves, knees, thighs, buttocks, genitals, waist, chest, back, shoulders, arms, etc. Once you have rested your entire body, spend a few minutes imagining yourself without judgment as: tremendously fat, skinny, tall, a midget, different races, the opposite sex, and pure light without form.

MORNING JOURNAL ENTRY

Write one sentence each about five to ten things in your life that are positive.

TODAY'S THINGS TO DO INSTEAD OF BINGEING

1. Remember the money you saved yesterday by not buying binge food? Think of an enjoyable way to spend it!
2. Start a list of everything and everyone that you love.
3. Work with diligence on your study project.
4. Review past options.

HOMEWORK: DAY 5

1. Write a physical description of yourself. Include what you

saw in the mirror on Day 3 when you studied your face and your hands, skin complexion and texture, hair, legs, etc. Who do you look like? What are some judgments you've made about your body? Do you wish that there were differences? What are they? Are they reasonable or even possible? Do you think other people make these same judgments about themselves?

2. Buy a mass market magazine. When you get home, go through the ads, articles, and photos. Tear out everything that promotes thinness or body change. Include thin models, advertisements that appeal to weight loss customers, "beautifying" products like cosmetics, or procedures like plastic surgery. How much of the magazine is left? Reflect on the economics and message of the medium in your journal. What would happen if all women loved their bodies just as they are? Tear the junk pile to shreds, while you *think lovely thoughts*.

3. Whenever you have a negative thought today, write it down, then tear up the paper. Replace the thought with a positive one!

4. Review the plan for Day 9 when you will be going on an all-day excursion. You may have to do some rearranging of your schedule and planning ahead, so start today. Contact a friend to accompany you.

5. Allow yourself a small dessert tonight, even if it is just one bite. Do not obsess about it, merely select and eat it as a reward for your efforts to end bulimia. Do not count calories. If you begin to even think negative thoughts after eating your dessert, immediately stop what you are doing and write in your journal. Then spend time stretching, going for a walk, or using another option.

GOOD NIGHT

Words, whether spoken or thought, have tremendous power. The way that we verbalize something is how we perceive it. If negative words are used, negative feelings surface. You may have gotten used to thinking of yourself as bulimic, worthless, unlovable, or unattractive. You must change those thoughts. You are *not a bulimic,* you are a worthwhile person of intrinsic beauty who *is recovering from bulimia.*

❧❦ DAY 6 ❧❦

I can accept support from others

We hope you had sweet dreams from your lovely thoughts of yesterday. Keep practicing and looking on the bright side.

THOUGHT FOR THE DAY

I can accept support from others.

Getting support does not mean only having horribly serious talks. A support relationship can be fun for both people. By asking someone to help you in recovery, you are being honest, respecting that person's point-of-view, and deepening the bonds of friendship. What could be better than that? You have many new experiences from this program alone. Share them!

THE MORNING WARM-UP

Loosen up with a quick, five minute stretch, followed by a long, hot shower. If you have body oil, splash it on!

TODAY'S THINGS TO DO INSTEAD OF BINGEING

1. Talk to a neighbor. Even casual conversation can distract you from bingeing.

2. Pamper your pet with fresh water, a bath, brush, or walk.

3. Go to a nursery, buy something, and plant it!

4. Collect some of your most meaningful possessions and make a little "shrine" for yourself. Use seashells, letters, photos, candles, a book, anything that is indicative of your personality. Add to this any day for support.

5. Consult your own list and pick one of the first three ideas.

HOMEWORK: DAY 6

1. Review your support list and pick one local person. Tell them that you have something important to talk about tonight, and also ask them to go with you to a movie. Watching a video or television is okay as a second choice. Meet at least an hour or two before the show starts to have enough time to talk about your recovery process. Follow that with the movie and perhaps a walk or a cup of coffee afterwards! If you or they have a previous commitment tonight, schedule this activity for the first available night. Make plans now!

2. Make a list of 5-10 myths and 5-10 rules that you may want to change. A myth may be something like, "Skinny people are happier." A rule may be something like, "I can't eat ice cream at night, because I'll gain weight."

3. What progress have you made with investigating therapy? Try at least an introductory session. We push this strongly because there are many skillful and knowledgeable professionals treating eating disorders. Find one who can help you!

GOOD NIGHT

We hope you took the risk to reach out today. That's such an important step. If you didn't talk to someone today, you've got homework to do! We bet that you are a pretty likable person after all! Of the hundreds of people who have confessed their bulimia to us—we are sometimes the first ones told—each one has been sensitive, sincere, and usually able to joke. Great qualities! Incidentally, did you watch a movie? Was it as entertaining as your conversation with your support person?

🏵 DAY 7 🏵

Peace of Mind

Today you will finish the first week of this program to stop bingeing. Think about it for a moment. Have your binges decreased this week? Have you practiced new coping skills that you particularly like? Most of the course emphasis so far has been on getting to know yourself better and to start reaching out. Next week, we will encourage you to interact even more. However, today you deserve to take it a little easier. Still, you must not slack off on your commitment to doing the homework, nor should you binge.

THOUGHT FOR THE DAY

I deserve rest and relaxation.

Many bulimics are high-achievers and feel guilty if they are not being productive. Life is not a race or contest; everyone needs to kick back at times. If bingeing has been a way for you to unwind or be entertained, you need new outlets. You are not just a "human doing," you are also a "human being." Allow yourself to just be.

THE MORNING WARM-UP

Use the progressive relaxation technique from Day 5. Today, though, when you are in that state of deep physical relaxation, visualize a special place. This can be somewhere that you know well or an imaginary spot. Put yourself there by seeing the sights, hearing the sounds, smelling the scents, and feeling your entire being in that restful scene.

TODAY'S THINGS TO DO INSTEAD OF BINGEING

1. Listen to or play music. Can you let go of tension and relax?
2. Flush what would have been your binge food down the disposal. Do you see the irony?
3. Try gardening, taking a slow walk, doing a yoga class, or going for a drive just to see the sights.
4. Repeat this morning's relaxation, but outside in the fresh air, and return to your special place.

HOMEWORK: DAY 7

1. Write or call someone you love. We recommend seeking out a person whom you have not seen for a long time but care for, such as a childhood friend or relative.
2. Read the plan for Day 9, and make any necessary preparations for that day's activities.
3. Recovery is not an event, it is a process, and an imperfect

one at that. There will be days when you slip, feel discouraged, or want to give up. Can you accept that you are always doing the best you can at any given moment? Even a setback is the best you could do sometimes. Write yourself a letter of encouragement and forgiveness for past setbacks.

4. Work on your study project.

5. Today, speak less. Try to reflect more on your inner thoughts. Silence is wonderful!

GOOD NIGHT

We suggest that you get to bed early tonight and enjoy a long sleep. Congratulations on sticking to the program for a week. That is an amazing feat!

ᘓᙦ *DAY 8* ᘓᙦ

Love Day!

Today is "Love Day" and you're going to love it! Last week we concentrated on inner growth. This week we will expand our horizons to include people, places, and outside experiences.

THOUGHT FOR THE DAY

I love me.

If you think no one loves you, that your parents didn't, your friends don't, and you're sure that the "right" guy or gal won't, how can you love yourself? You must realize that you are the source of love. Love doesn't come from "out there;" it comes from within you.

THE MORNING WARM-UP

Take a sensual shower or hot bath. Don't just soak or wash but massage your muscles. Appreciate the sensuality of your skin. Touch yourself with a lover's embrace. If your situation permits, share this experience.

SHORT JOURNAL ENTRY

Write your definition of "love." In what ways can you bring more love into your life?

TODAY'S THINGS TO DO INSTEAD OF BINGEING

1. Let's review a few from last week: exercise, soak food, beat up a pillow, get away, drink water, read your joke book. Have you tried these yet?

2. Take a round-trip bus ride anywhere. Observe the people on the bus; practice seeing each of them through loving eyes. Do not eat on this trip!

3. Try prayer.

4. Go to a lovely spot away from home, like a park, the beach, a particular tree or grove, or overlooking a beautiful scene. Close your eyes, count your breaths, and relax.

HOMEWORK: DAY 8

1. Do a good deed. Some possibilities: visit a nursing home and give of yourself by talking to an elderly person, baby-sit for a friend with small children, visit someone and help them clean or cook, offer your services to a non-profit organization, etc. Don't just call or think about it. This is the main assignment today, go

somewhere and do it!

2. Tell someone you love them and why. This can be done in writing.

3. Continue to work on these earlier assignments: arranging for professional therapy and contacting people from your support list.

4. Have you lined up someone to join you on Day 9?

5. Throughout the day, look at your reflection in different mirrors and windows. Does your mood depend on what you see? Think about it.

6. To elicit feelings of love, listen to a favorite old song or piece of music, look through a scrapbook or photo album, write or call a friend you haven't seen in years.

GOOD NIGHT

Everyday can be a "Love Day" if you practice. As we said before, love is not something that comes from outside of you. As we wrote this book, feelings of love generated the words. Doing good deeds, helping others, feeling positive about ourselves, these make us feel more "full" than food ever can.

❧❧ *DAY 9* ❧❧

It Takes All Kinds to Make a World

Invite someone to join you in today's activities which revolve around role playing. Most of the time, we get too caught up in our identities and our own particular roles, acting in ways to please our parents, bosses, teachers, and friends. What about you? Do you live for others with little regard for your own feelings? Do you want to be thin to please a lover, parent, or society? Who makes judgments about you? Is it okay to be different from the norm? Don't be afraid of what people think; be fearless!

THOUGHT FOR THE DAY

It's all right to be different.

Today, you will be! Create a new identity for yourself and act it out! You don't have to be someone exotic—you can be what you consider to be a "normal" person. Obviously, continuing this masquerade all day can be difficult, but do your best. Be that person as much as possible, and use this "distance" to get to know yourself better. This can be fun as well as revealing. Of course, *you must choose not to be bulimic.*

THE MORNING WARM-UP

As you know by reading today's plan, you are going to pretend to be someone else today. Wash your hair and fix it how the other person would wear it—maybe with a scarf, curls, parted in the middle, etc. Dress as this person would dress. If you are usually casual, perhaps you'll wear more formal clothing. If you usually wear makeup, maybe this person won't. As you "put on your costume," begin to assume the new identity.

MORNING JOURNAL ENTRY

Write about the person you are pretending to be. What are your likes and dislikes? What's your background? What special talents do you have? What do you like to eat? Make your description interesting and complete. Become that person for the day.

TODAY'S THINGS TO DO INSTEAD OF BINGEING

1. The person you're pretending to be doesn't binge!

2. Use your support person.

3. Go to a busy intersection and people-watch. Notice how different everyone is.

4. Buy a national newspaper or magazine. How many thin people are shown in pictures or ads? How many weight loss methods can you count? Rip it to shreds!

HOMEWORK: DAY 9

1. Today you will be going on an all-day—or at least a few hours—excursion. If it is absolutely impossible for you to take the day off, then substitute this day for the earliest one possible.

2. You've been instructed to read today's lesson and to invite a friend to join you. If you are doing it with a friend, warn them in advance that you are going to be "in character" and he or she might want to be, too. It may sound crazy and you might be slightly embarrassed to suggest it, but both of you will have fun.

3. Leave your usual surroundings by going on an outing consistent with your new character. Maybe you are an artist and can visit a museum. Maybe you are a surfer and will hit the beach! Bring anything that the "pretend you" would bring. Even introduce yourself to people along the way as this other person. Have fun. Go with it!

4. If your character is more reckless than you might usually be, still use good judgment.

5. When you return home, sit quietly for at least five minutes and relax. After that, write in your journal. As helpful as it is to get away, it is crucial to maintain your positive feelings and actions upon return.

6. Write a journal entry: What aspects of your "make-believe" character would you like to keep for your own? Which aspects of "the real you" never changed?

GOOD NIGHT

Wherever you go, you can carry your old baggage with you or leave it behind—your choice!

𝒲𝒞 *DAY 10* 𝒲𝒞

Assert yourself!

Yesterday, we asked you to try being someone else. Now it's time to enjoy being who you are. People with bulimia are afraid to express their true selves. They hold back feelings and hide behind their food problems. They may have trouble actually knowing who they are or what they feel, but we are working to change that. Today, we want to help you get to know yourself better.

THOUGHT FOR THE DAY

I can assert myself!

Expose your feelings, opinions, and real self. It's okay if people don't always agree with you or if you don't always agree with them. There are times when you must say "no" and set your boundaries. This may mean choosing some different friends or living situations. The important thing is that you be true to yourself!

THE MORNING WARM-UP

Have a good, long (15-30 minutes) stretch and (optional) exercise workout.

TODAY'S THINGS TO DO INSTEAD OF BINGEING

1. Express a strong opinion. For example, write a television network to complain about offensive programming or advertising.

2. Say "NO!" out loud to bulimia.

3. Aggressively hammer nails, chop wood, or beat the stuffing out of a pillow.

4. Call a friend and share with each other your hopes and dreams for the future.

5. Take cans of food from your pantry or old clothes from your closet and donate them to a homeless shelter.

HOMEWORK: DAY 10

1. List 10 character traits you like about yourself.

2. Draw a self-portrait. Use a photo of yourself or look in the mirror. It doesn't have to be a work of art!

3. Talk or write to a family member about your recovery from bulimia. This can be the same person you've spoken with before, or a different relative.

4. Make a list of ways in which you can say "no" to someone without hurting their feelings. Perhaps start with an "I" phrase, such as "I'm feeling a little unsure how to put this. . . but I don't like what you are doing," or "I hope you can understand my point of view. . . but I'd rather not go with you today." Practicing saying what you are feeling makes it easier when the time comes.

5. Work on your study project. This has been something we

have not said much about, other than to do it. If you have gotten into this project, it is already giving you great rewards.

GOOD NIGHT

Ten days is a long time to follow a regime such as ours. Congratulate yourself on getting this far, regardless of whether or not you've binged. As you lie in bed, feel the tension drift out of your body. The more time you spend away from bulimia, the better you will feel.

🦋 *DAY 11* 🦋

Getting What You Want

If wanting to binge has been your top priority, you have ignored a world of wonderful possibilities. Ask small children what they want to be when they grow up, and you might hear answers like astronaut, the richest person in the world, movie star, President, or professional athlete. No one says, "I want to be bulimic." Now that you have decided that you *don't* want to be bulimic, what *do* you want?

THOUGHT FOR THE DAY

I can get what I want.

We already know that you do not want to be bulimic anymore; but what *do* you want? There are "wants" of a physical nature: I want a new car, I want to go on vacation, or I want to *look* attractive. There are also "wants" of an inner nature: I want to be happy, I want to love myself, or I want to *feel* attractive.

Think about what *you* want.

THE MORNING WARM-UP

Go for a walk or gentle jog of about 15 minutes. Be sure to stretch first. Do not run a race!

TODAY'S THINGS TO DO INSTEAD OF BINGEING

1. Have a meal with a support person. Choose foods that you would really enjoy eating. Leave some on your plate and express thanks for the meal.

2. Go somewhere tourists go. Buy a souvenir.

3. Instead of bingeing, give yourself a treat. Do #2 of today's homework.

4. Write these words 20 times in your notebook, "I want to quit bulimia!"

HOMEWORK: DAY 11

1. List 25 "I Wants!" including things you want to own, do, and feel. Separate them into short-term and long-term. Pick three and make plans to work towards or achieve them soon.

2. If you think you are ready, treat yourself to a piece of candy or favorite "forbidden" food and eat it in a special place. Perhaps have a support person with you. Eating in moderation is tremendously challenging, but rewarding on many different levels.

3. Buy yourself something with money you would have spent on food.

4. Make an appointment with a therapist today, if you have not already done so.

5. Work on your study project.

GOOD NIGHT

You've started to focus on some of your "wants." These are much healthier thoughts than obsessing about bingeing. Keep thinking about positive goals. Believe in yourself. You *can* get some of the things you want. Also, now you are more than halfway through this program. Keep going! Get even more into it!

〰 DAY 12 〰

Size Acceptance

The pressure to be thin hurts everyone. Fat people are discriminated against and thin people are afraid to be fat. Practically everyone believes that being thin is important and the vast majority dislike their bodies. This is a sad situation. Why can't we accept our bodies just as they are? We can.

THOUGHT FOR THE DAY

My goodness has nothing to do with my size or weight.

Who you are is more important than how you look. Thus far we have been encouraging you to love and trust your inner self. Now is the time to start accepting your outer self. Your worth is not based on a number on a scale. You can be loved and loving with a body of any size or shape. That is far more important than thinness.

THE MORNING WARM-UP

Study your body in a mirror. Start by putting aside your desires to be thinner, have different hair or complexion, be taller or shorter, etc. Affirm that your body is perfectly all right the way it is. While you are observing, remember that no one has an "ideal" body, not even the models in the magazines. Imagine a lover who desires you exactly as you see your reflection.

TODAY'S THINGS TO DO INSTEAD OF BINGEING

1. Gentle, stretching exercise; then a quick, short walk.

2. Make a list of 25 good things your body does for you, like making it possible to dance, feel the warmth of a fire, or build a snow man.

3. Try fitting your body into a space that is too small, such as under a chair or desk. This is the type of prison you have made for yourself with bulimia.

4. Clean out your closet and donate what doesn't fit to a thrift store. Go out and buy some clothes that fit well to replace them.

5. Try standing on your head using a pillow and a wall.

HOMEWORK: DAY 12

1. List some "happy couples" you know. Are they in love? Do you think they have a good relationship? Do they have "ideal" bodies?

2. Write a description of a planet where your body is the ideal. How does that make you feel? What do you feel towards the other people whose bodies are not this ideal? Compassion, superiority, sympathy, love? What about a planet where every person loved their body exactly the way it was, with unique lumps, bumps, and curves? It is possible for every shape and size to be beautiful in its own way!

3. Go to a shopping area—maybe the same place you're get-

ting clothing that fits—and observe people. What do they look like? Does anyone have an "ideal" body? Do smaller people seem happier than larger people? Are people eating-on-the-run? Do they seem happy? Does anyone judge your appearance? Record some observations and thoughts.

4. Throughout the day notice how you hold yourself. See if you slouch or are upright, if you smile or frown, if you look at people's eyes or look away, etc. What do your body signs say about how you feel about yourself?

GOOD NIGHT

Children in elementary school are already concerned about their weight and appearance, but there was a time earlier than that when they were joyful about their bodies. Think of a toddler thrilled at learning to walk, a baby sucking happily on its toes, or how fun it was to take a bubble bath. Remember the wonderful smell of baked cookies before you began to worry about calories? Get in touch with the innocent time of your life when you loved your body.

〰 DAY 13 〰

Small Steps Add Up!

You have made a strong commitment to ending your bulimia, which is obvious if you are still following this program or are using parts of it. Keep paving the way for your future with baby steps. The rewards of recovery can be found in the process as well as the goal. In other words, working on your recovery can make you feel just as good as being recovered.

THOUGHT FOR THE DAY

I can make small changes with big results!

Some aspects of your life will have to change in order to support health and wellness. Fill your days with more positive energy and make even small adjustments to your environment and routine to help you get stronger in your battle to beat bulimia. Notice the details. They add up.

THE MORNING WARM-UP

Do a music appreciation activity. Some ideas: listen with headphones to your favorite song, play an instrument, sing, or dance. Listen to a tape or CD of nature sounds.

SHORT JOURNAL ENTRY

Write about what you've learned in your study project, then reflect on your feelings about it, such as: accomplishment, intellectual fulfillment, stimulation, interest, etc. If you haven't gotten into a study project, write about what other activities or hesitations have kept you from doing it.

TODAY'S THINGS TO DO INSTEAD OF BINGEING

1. If you have not already done so, get rid of your scale. Write it a goodbye letter and run over it with your car!

2. Put an unsigned classified ad in the personals column of your newspaper that says, "I am quitting bulimia! I placed this ad instead of bingeing. I am proud of myself!"

3. Put a picture of yourself in a spot you would normally reserve for a loved one. Place fresh flowers beside it.

4. Donate binge money to charity.

5. Buy colored, sticky stars to put on your calendar for every day that you do not binge.

HOMEWORK: DAY 13

1. List 10-20 things which maintain your bulimia and brainstorm alternatives. Notice the environment—the usual times or places you binge, friends who are negative influences, rituals and habits that have you trapped, etc. For example: If you binge while driving to work, you can (a) take a bus or car pool, (b) not take food with you on the drive, or (c) listen to a book on tape to change the routine.

2. Tell someone you love them. Look in the mirror and tell yourself! You're someone!

3. Work on your study project and complete unfinished homework from previous days.

4. Clean up your desk or work area. Organize your supplies and make some small changes. Perhaps buy a new address book to accommodate your new support system, or buy a new blotter or ream of colored paper instead of white. Add flowers!

GOOD NIGHT

Every time you do not binge may seem like a small step, but its effects are enormous. Every success is a gift to your true self. You are worth it.

❧ *DAY 14* ❧

Count your blessings

Despite the pain in our lives, we are fortunate in many ways. One only has to look at the world's victims of war and disease to realize that other people have big problems of their own. Even people you pass on the street have hardships and pain that you might not see. Today, give thanks for the good things that do exist in your life and for the possibilities that are yet to come.

THOUGHT FOR THE DAY

Notice miracles.

Small miracles happen everyday, which you usually do not notice. They can be as simple as the way you feel when you see the smile on a child's face, or as stupendous as meeting your soul mate at a shopping mall. Contemplate some of the everyday miracles you've experienced and be open to the ones that are yet to come.

THE MORNING WARM-UP

Spend 20 minutes in quiet time. You can use any of the techniques that have been suggested in this book, or sit comfortably in a quiet place, close your eyes, and silently count to ten. When finished, count to ten again, and again, and over and over. Let your mind go.

SHORT JOURNAL ENTRY

Write a message of gratitude to anyone who once did something of special kindness for you. Send or keep in your journal.

TODAY'S THINGS TO DO INSTEAD OF BINGEING

1. Go to a place of worship, take a walk in nature.

2. Write a letter of forgiveness, which you may or may not send, to someone who has wronged you. Forgiveness does not justify or condone the actions of the person, but is an act of the heart that sets you free.

3. Put your binge food in a shopping bag and carry it to any public trash can. Walk there with purpose and throw the bag away.

4. Consult your list of successful options and pick one.

HOMEWORK: DAY 14

1. Make a list of the ways in which bulimia has taken care of you. Then, write it a thank-you note, and tell it that you are saying goodbye.

2. Write your definition of "God" and what that means to you.

3. Get in about an hour of fun, healthy exercise. Choose something outside of your home—walking in a beautiful place, hitting tennis balls with a friend, going for a bike ride, etc.

4. Do one act of random kindness today. It might be something as simple as opening a door for someone, donating to a charity, or spending time with someone who needs attention.

GOOD NIGHT

Imagine the scope of the universe. How many people have lived before you and will after you're gone? Think of how small you are in the scheme of things, how small your problems are. Finally, try to feel that all of the universe and all of humanity exists only inside of your heart and mind. Be thankful to be alive.

❦ *DAY 15* ❦

Looking at Your Family

For better or worse—or most likely somewhere in between—your family has had a profound influence on you. Genetics causes you to look like them. From them, you have learned how to communicate, problem solve, and handle feelings. Your belief and value systems are also closely related to your role within the family. There is no escaping your family's influence on you, but there is understanding and making peace with it.

THOUGHT FOR THE DAY

I can be my own person.

Even though we just mentioned your family's influence, you are not the same as them. You may share some experiences and traits, but you have a life all of your own. Your journey is unique. Your era, friends, mentors, lessons, path, and heart are completely different from theirs. Celebrate your uniqueness!

THE MORNING WARM-UP

Take another long look at yourself in a mirror. What features and body parts came from which parents and grandparents? Whose eyes, hair, nose, and hips do you have? Look through photos of your parents, grandparents, siblings, and self at various ages. How similar is your shape and size to theirs? Try to accept that you cannot change your genetics. If you don't like looking like the rest of your family, perhaps you should think about why that is.

SHORT JOURNAL ENTRY

Write about one happy time spent with your family. Why did you pick that memory?

TODAY'S THINGS TO DO INSTEAD OF BINGEING

1. Diagram your family tree, going back at least as far as your grandparents.

2. Punch, kick, and yell at an inanimate object (like a pillow or punching bag) as if it is a family member who makes you mad.

3. Call a loving relative just to talk.

4. Make a list of the things your family does that provoke you to binge. For instance, they might appear angry or treat you like you are invisible.

HOMEWORK: DAY 15

1. Notice that Day 19 may require scheduling in advancing or swapping days. Prepare for that if necessary.

2. Answer the following questions:
   - Do you have a role within your family?
   - If you are the firstborn, are you expected to be more of a parent than a child?
   - Are you the dreamer, scapegoat, baby, or peacemaker?
   - Reflect how your role has limited your interactions with people inside and outside of the family.

3. Confront your feelings about family members. Choose one member of your family, and write about a difficult moment in the following manner:
   - During your lifetime, recall one time when this person said or did something that made you feel bad.

- How did you react?
- Why has this event stuck with you?
- What do you wish you had said or done at the time?
- What could he or she have said or done to convey their message in a more positive manner?
- Could the two of you communicate about it when it happened?
- Is it worth talking about now?
- Have you forgiven them? Can you? (See yesterday's "Things to Do" #2).

4. Look at the supportive role your family has played by answering these questions:

- Which family members have supported you?
- How do they support you now?
- Are they doing their best?
- Which others would you like to be more involved with your life?
- Can you accept that some may be unable to be there for you in the way you'd like them to be?
- Is there anything obvious *you* can do to improve your relationships with your family?

GOOD NIGHT

Maybe you were fortunate enough to have parents who lovingly tucked you into bed at night. If so, think about that experience tonight. If not, imagine what it would feel like to be a small child with a seemingly-omniscient parent who unconditionally loves you. This may not be like the parents you had, but try to feel that kind of love emanating from within yourself. Ultimately, we all have to grow up and learn to parent ourselves.

❧❧ *DAY 16* ❧❧

Embrace the arts.

Artists of all kinds often feel connected to a higher power through their art. Some speak of the act of painting a picture or composing a song as if they themselves were the brush or instrument in the hands of a greater presence. When you look at a work of art or hear a masterpiece of music, you can feel the source of inspiration. Let's get in touch with those feelings today.

THOUGHT FOR THE DAY

I will see the beauty around me and within me.

Art is a reflection of the beauty that is everywhere to be seen or an inner vision that needs to be expressed. Some artists turn their pain and suffering into magnificence. Look around; look within. See the beauty.

THE MORNING WARM-UP

Listen to one of your most favorite songs. Play it over again. Sing it in the shower.

SHORT JOURNAL ENTRY

Try to articulate what it is that appeals to you about a favorite painter or painting. Be visual and descriptive.

TODAY'S THINGS TO DO INSTEAD OF BINGEING

1. Get some washable markers or inexpensive stage makeup and draw on your face. Give yourself a mustache or clown face.

Looking like that, how can you possibly take yourself so seriously as to binge?

2. If there is someone from your original, proposed support list whom you've resisted telling about your recovery from bulimia, talk to them today or write in your notebook about why you haven't contacted them.

3. Make random designs on a piece of paper or buy a coloring book and spend time coloring in the spaces.

4. Look through an art book one page at a time until you can pick one or two favorites.

HOMEWORK: DAY 16

1. Spend at least two to three hours beginning a two-day project. Choose now whether to work with art or music.

a. If you selected *art*, your assignment is to create a painting based on a photograph, landscape, still life, or portrait. Use any media. Today, begin by collecting the materials you will need, and pick a subject. If you are having difficulty deciding what to paint, do a self-portrait or arrange a few mundane articles on a table and do a still life. Make several sketches before you do the actual painting, which will be worked on tomorrow, as well. Attempt to finish this painting during these two days, but take an extra day if you need it. Feel free to paint in any style and try to not be concerned about the final picture.

b. If you selected *music*, your assignment is to compose a song with or without words, for any instrument or instruments, and in any style. If this is new to you, work first at finding a central melody. Try a few different keys until you hit upon something that strikes a chord within you. If you get blocked, rely upon a few basic progressions and take it from there. You can either write sheet music or tape record your efforts as you experiment. If you draft a few quick fragments, you can choose from them tomorrow as you further develop the song.

2. Tell a support person about the art or music project you've undertaken. Express any fears about not doing a good-enough job, and acknowledge that the process of creation is more important than the final product.

3. Purchase a CD or tape of music you think will inspire you. If you have difficulty choosing one, try movie soundtracks or a selection of arias by Puccini, the opera composer.

GOOD NIGHT

One of life's great rewards is leaving a legacy, such as a work of art, and everyone does that in one way or another. In fact, you have an effect on all of the people you meet without even realizing the significance of your interactions. Think a little about what you might want to leave behind to the benefit of others. It is probably a much greater gift than you think.

❦❧ DAY 17 ❦❧

You are not alone.

Millions of people suffer from eating disorders. More than 100,000 throughout the world have read this book, and some are working through this program right now, at the same time as you! Although you are anonymous from one another—and we won't meet most of you either—understand that we all share a deep and meaningful connection. There is support out there even from people you don't know.

THOUGHT FOR THE DAY

I'm not alone in my recovery.

In addition to the inspiration of those you don't know, appreciate the support you've been getting from those close to you. Be thankful and respectful.

THE MORNING WARM-UP

While in the shower or in front of a mirror, give a pep talk to an imagined dear one who is working on their recovery from bulimia. Reach into the heart of your own experience to get through to them. *Speak out loud!*

SHORT JOURNAL ENTRY

Write about someone who has overcome an obstacle. You might personally know them and know their story or use an historical figure.

TODAY'S THINGS TO DO INSTEAD OF BINGEING

1. Visit an animal shelter, pet store, or zoo.

2. Look up bulimia on the Internet. You can start at our web page, www.bulimia.com, which has links to many other sites. Perhaps try a chat room where there are other people who are struggling with an eating disorder.

3. Make up an imaginary support group. Who would you include and why? These can be real, imagined, fictitious, or historical people.

4. Eat a meal with a support person.

HOMEWORK: DAY 17

1. Try to complete your art or music project today.

2. Get a biography or someone's personal story of recovery that particularly interests you and which will make you feel less alone. For example, Lindsey's book *Full Lives: Women Who Have Freed Themselves from Food & Weight Obsession* has over a dozen contributors whose stories may reflect your own. Read it slowly so that you will still be reading when this three-week program has finished. Think of your book as a transitional object that represents recovery work that will continue on after we've stopped providing you with homework.

3. Make an effort to locate a recovered mentor. Try a local hospital that has an eating disorder unit, a therapist who specializes in eating problems, or a organization with support groups (see Resources) who might be able to help you with this.

GOOD NIGHT

On a dark, clear night away from city lights, the sky is filled with stars. You know what it looks like. Imagine the stars as people who have already recovered from an eating disorder. They are shining down on you with their energy and love.

❧❧ *DAY 18* ❧❧

Living in the Now!

When you think too much about the future or the past, you miss your life as it is happening right now. Bulimia is a way of avoiding the present, because if you're not in the midst of a binge, you are either planning the next binge or feeling guilty over the last one. Live in the moment.

THOUGHT FOR THE DAY

Live in the moment.

Practice this by concentrating on what you are doing at all times. Have an awareness of the world around you. If you notice your mind wandering, bring it back to the present. Do this with the verbal reminder, "Live in the moment."

THE MORNING WARM-UP

Observe your typical morning hygiene with an awareness of the moment. For example, as you wash your face, do it thoroughly using warm water, soap, and a washcloth. Scrub the pores deeply. Rinse completely, being sure to remove all of the soap. Gently dry with a clean, soft towel. Perform these tasks with a mindful purpose and focus only on the task at hand.

SHORT JOURNAL ENTRY

Write about the first thing that comes into your mind. Come up with any topic and just go with it.

TODAY'S THINGS TO DO INSTEAD OF BINGEING

1. Sign up for something physically and emotionally challenging, like a ropes course, Outward Bound excursion, or river rafting trip. If you are afraid of heights, walking over a tall bridge is an act of bravery that will keep you from thinking about anything else.

2. Pick up trash at a park or beach.

3. Carefully look at a work of art. Why is it considered art? How does it affect you? What styles and techniques did the artist use? Be analytic and opinionated.

4. Drink two glasses of water.

HOMEWORK: DAY 18

1. Throughout the day you will have many types of feelings (anger, wonderment, resentment, joy, etc.); try to put a name to them as they occur. For example, if you are feeling angry, notice that and say to yourself, "I'm feeling angry." As you get the chance, list these feelings in your notebook and read over the list at the end of the day.

2. Visit someone with small children or observe a day care center. Watch how kids are present in the moment. Also, observe some animals. See how an ant follows its path with purpose, a cow merely eats and rests, and a cat does what it wants when it wants. None are concerned with the past or future. Take a cue from them about how to live in the moment.

3. Do something fun today that requires your constant attention, like playing tennis, chess, or a musical instrument.

4. Meditate for at least 20 minutes using one of the techniques described earlier or one of your own choosing. Try not to let your mind wander.

GOOD NIGHT

You can think about the past, but *right now* is what is real. This moment is what you're experiencing. Let go of the past; old concepts don't work anymore. Don't dwell on the future. We don't know what awaits—other than that there will be surprises. Make the most of every day.

〰 *DAY 19* 〰

Listen to Your Inner Voice

Within you is a tremendous source of love and wisdom. By quieting the mind of negative self-talk and unnecessary chatter, you will begin to experience this inner source. Today, do not speak unless you must. Avoid unnecessary input like newspapers, television, and radio, though peaceful music is okay. Reading or writing (except letters or Internet chat) is fine. Fill the day with contemplation and silence, and listen for your inner voice.

THOUGHT FOR THE DAY

Silence is golden.

Have you ever gone a day without speaking? It is a challenging and rewarding endeavor. When you are quiet, your mind will also get quieter. Without constant chatter, you will feel more peaceful and content. Then you will know why silence is precious.

THE MORNING WARM-UP

Reread the sections "Spiritual Pursuits" and "Changing Your Mind" in Chapter Five (pages 162-170), which sets today's tone.

SHORT JOURNAL ENTRY

To reaffirm the goals for this course, write down each of the

"Thought for the Day" expressions from the past 18 days. Think about each one.

TODAY'S THINGS TO DO INSTEAD OF BINGEING

1. Pray
2. Meditate
3. Climb into bed and read.
4. Do a cleanup project, such as sorting through a closet, pulling weeds, or scrubbing a floor.
5. Stare at a lit candle or flames in a fireplace.

HOMEWORK: DAY 19

1. Take quiet time for 20-30 minutes at least twice today using any of the relaxation techniques described earlier or another that you have learned.

2. Can you remember when your intuition about a situation was perfectly correct? Maybe you knew exactly what someone was going to say during a conversation or have felt "right on" about a decision, perhaps knowing that you should do this program. Your intuition is a powerful voice—be quiet and listen!

3. Go somewhere to stare at flowing water. This can be a river, lake, fountain, etc. Spend at least 30 minutes listening to the sound of the water and let your mind wander. If negative thoughts arise, ease them away with an affirmation.

4. Write an imaginary, heartfelt acceptance speech. It can be for something that exists, like an Academy Award or Most Valuable Player, or something you make up, like Best Recovering Bulimic or Most Sensitive Person.

GOOD NIGHT

We think of you with great love and respect. Truly, as we write we feel your presence as if you are in the room with us. We share a consciousness that resonates through our inner voices. It is compassionate and wants only what is best for us.

❦ *DAY 20* ❦

Think ahead.

Whether you've stuck to our three-week program or are just reading through it for ideas, you need to be thinking about the future. How do you want your life to be and what can you do to make it that way?

THOUGHT FOR THE DAY

My life really is better without bulimia!

On Day 1 we asked you to repeat this thought over and over. Today, you can say it with more conviction because, hopefully, you've experienced some peace from bulimia during these past three weeks. Keep repeating this phrase from now on, even after your bulimia is a distant memory.

THE MORNING WARM-UP

Celebrate your successes for the past weeks. First off, give yourself three cheers (such as "Hip, hip, hooray"). Next, play inspirational or favorite music and dance and sing along. Finally, loudly proclaim "My life really is better without bulimia!"

SHORT JOURNAL ENTRY

Write about the longest period of time you've gone without bingeing since becoming bulimic. How did you feel about your life during that break? How did you stop yourself from bingeing? Do you believe you can go longer and longer with practice?

TODAY'S THINGS TO DO INSTEAD OF BINGEING

1. Read all of your "Short Journal Entries."
2. If you haven't already done so, make a "shrine" for yourself with your picture, flowers, and other special objects.
3. Write lyrics to the song "Bye Bye Bulimia."
4. Pick one day at random and do the second option on that day's list, whatever it is!

HOMEWORK: DAY 20

1. What are your goals for the next few days, weeks, months, and years? Make lists or a timeline.
2. Make a list of at 20-25 "B" activities. Essential "A" activities include eat, sleep, work, wash, etc. "B" activities are those that are not essential, but are enriching and enjoyable, like listening to music, exercising, going places, reading, etc. In the future, refer to this list and do at least a couple of "B" activities every day.
3. Read through your notebook.
4. Complete unfinished homework.
5. Final reminder: Try some form of professional therapy.

GOOD NIGHT

Not everyone who reads this book will do or even attempt to do this program. Many people may be attracted to the title, "A

Three-Week Program to Stop Bingeing," but will shy away from actually *doing* anything. Regardless of whether or not you have binged, if you have followed this course fairly faithfully, you have accomplished a great feat. Think back to some of the fun moments, happy thoughts, and special places. Pleasant dreams.

🌾 DAY 21 🌾

Graduation Day!

Today is Graduation Day, and you should be quite proud of yourself. Hum "Pomp and Circumstance" (the graduation tune) to yourself all day. As with most education, graduating means new challenges, independence, and some uncertainty. By doing this program, you have progressed far in your recovery, and now we ask you to reach ever farther. Bulimia will get more and more distant from your thoughts and consciousness as long as you keep making an effort.

THOUGHT FOR THE DAY

I have accomplished something big!

Let's summarize some of the things that you have done in this course. You've set goals, taken initiative, examined feelings about your family, laughed, learned something new, been honest and open with others, relaxed, looked at your values, identified wants, made affirmations, practiced eating without bingeing, and expressed love. Have pride; your horizons are limitless.

THE MORNING WARM-UP

Read through the past 20 Morning Warm-ups, and remember your experiences doing them. Do these kinds of activities every morning. Today, repeat one that you particularly liked.

SHORT JOURNAL ENTRY

Write feedback to us about the three-week program. You do not have to send it, but may if you wish.

TODAY'S THINGS TO DO INSTEAD OF BINGEING

1. Visit a preschool. Watch the children. You, too, are starting fresh.
2. Put binge food in a bag and drive over it with your car.
3. Plant a tree in honor of your graduation.
4. Go somewhere with your journal and make a list of all the things you have done in the last three weeks to *not* binge.

HOMEWORK: DAY 21

We wouldn't make you do homework on graduation day! However, you must realize by now that you have to keep working every day on your continuing recovery. Even as you gently let go of your bulimia, you can embrace every day with the attitudes that we've encouraged—looking for solutions not problems, being positive, accepting support, resting when you need it, and loving yourself.

GOOD NIGHT

We're nostalgic writing this final message to you. We have shared our selves, hoping that you will be motivated in your recovery. Think of us cheering you on while you continue making progress. With all our hearts, we wish you love, happiness, and freedom from bulimia.

We'd like to hear from you!

Nothing has given us greater satisfaction or has touched our hearts more than the beautiful letters we have received from people who have read our books. You can write to us care of Gürze Books (B5), PO. Box 2238, Carlsbad, CA 92018.

CHAPTER 10

A Guide for Support Groups

Throughout the United States and Canada, ongoing support groups can often be located by contacting local treatment facilities, hospitals, therapists, women's centers, or college health or counseling centers. Overeaters Anonymous serves this function for many people. Additionally, the eating disorder organizations listed in the "Resources" section of this book may be able to help you find a group. Finally, there are eating disorders support groups on the Internet.

However, there is a chance that you will not be able to find a group in your area. So, we offer this guide which takes a group from conception through six meetings, with a framework for future sessions. *We strongly encourage you to find a professional to facilitate your group at some point,* but you can get started without one while you look for someone you like.

Note: These guidelines have been adopted for use by many professional therapists and self-led bulimia groups. Permission is hereby granted for this chapter to be duplicated for future use.

Forming the Group

As we said before, if no professionally-led groups are available in your area, use the guidelines in this section to start your own. This means gathering your courage and taking the initiative to search out members. Classified advertising in a college or local newspaper might get enough responses to fill a group. Here's how you might word the ad:

"Stop your binge/vomiting. Join a free bulimia support group. Forming now to start (the date). Confidential! Call (Your phone number)."

An advertisement such as this costs less than a binge, and the group can share the expense once it gets going. Run the ad a few times to get between 5 and 10 people. Another good way to advertise for members is to place leaflets on bulletin boards in office buildings or on college campuses. Neatly present the same basic information as above on a sheet which may be photocopied. You may want to include your phone number on tear-off tabs at the bottom.

Arrange for the first meeting to be held at a public facility, and after that, your responsibilities as leader are over.

Rules of the Group

The following is a basic framework for support groups, which is intended to maintain a balance of order and positive reinforcement for the participants. Professionally-led groups can dispense with most of these structural technicalities, but can still use the basic ideas and activities that follow in the six agendas.

At the first meeting, review the following rules:

1. Any of these rules may be changed by consensus of the group. Consensus means that everyone agrees or agrees not to stop the mutual decision of the others.

2. The underlying issue for most bulimics is not food; therefore, the following subjects should not monopolize the discussions: diets, food, bingeing, weight control, etc.

3. Each group will follow the same basic format: introduction and goals, discussion, exercises, and summary. The topics and exercises will be provided here.

4. At each meeting, different people must be appointed to the following jobs, which may be rotated:

- facilitator (group leader to introduce each topic and call on people to speak)
- time-keeper (to keep on schedule)
- gripe-control monitor (to interrupt anyone who is monopolizing the focus)

5. At the beginning of each meeting, the agenda will be reviewed and anyone who wants to add an item may do so.

6. One requirement of all group members is complete honesty.

7. No meeting shall end on a pessimistic or depressed note. If these conditions exist at the scheduled close, then a discussion or activity must be enacted to uplift the spirit of the group.

First Meeting Agenda

1. Review the rules of the group.

2. Appoint facilitator, time-keeper, and gripe-control monitor. These positions might not be necessary in professionally-led groups.

3. The facilitator reviews this agenda with the group, and agenda items are added. Approximate times are allocated for each item.

4. **Introduction:** Everyone in the group introduces themselves and explains why they have joined the group. Keep these introductions to a couple of minutes each.

5. **Discussion:** This meeting's topic is about the nature of support. To begin the discussion, each member of the group takes turns answering some of the following questions:

- Who has been supportive of your recovery, and what have they done that has been helpful?

- If anyone else knows about your bulimia, how did they react when they found out, and how did that make you feel?

- What are a few do's and don'ts you would recommend to someone in order to help you recover from bulimia?

- What will you offer to other members of the group to support them?

- After the circle is complete, the group can have an open discussion about some of the things that came out in the exercise. This is not to psychoanalyze each other, but to gain insight through each other's disclosures. (20-40 minutes).

6. **Exercise:** Relaxation! (15-20 minutes)

Everyone gets into a comfortable position, either sitting or lying down. One person talks the others through the exercise in a soothing, monotone voice, while the others relax with their eyes closed. Here is the exercise:

Take three deep breaths, inhaling, holding the breath, and exhaling, each to the count of ten (one-two-three...to ten inhaling, one-two-three...to ten holding, one-two-three...to ten exhaling). Afterwards, breathe normally. As you inhale, feel as though you are being filled with light; and as you exhale, empty yourself of stress. Feel your body relax. Concentrate on your toes, relax them. Continue this, relaxing your feet, ankles, calves, knees, etc., until every part of the body is mentioned. Feel yourself filled with light and health, goodness, purity, contentment, power, etc. Remain in this state for several minutes before slowly reviving.

7. **Summary:** The group needs to set a time and place for the next meeting. It can be as soon as tomorrow! Because this is a support group, a commitment needs to be made by the members to come to at least the next meeting, with the intention of coming to all six. Exchange phone numbers so that individuals can use each other for support outside of the group.

A Few Words About Your Progress: This first meeting may have been difficult for you. Opening up may not have been easy or even possible. Give yourself some time; it will get easier. Individual or group therapy, medical examinations, and other steps towards self-help that are suggested in this book need to be made in addition to the support group. In any case, stick to your commitment to getting better and remember that you make your own choices.

Second Meeting Agenda

1. If appropriate, appoint a new facilitator, time-keeper, and gripe-control monitor.

2. Review the guidelines of the group and agenda.

3. **Introduction:** "I wish...," "I want...," and "I am..."

Everyone takes a few minutes to think about their answers to the above sentences within the context of recovery issues. Then, they take turns giving answers for "I wish . . ." until everyone has had a chance to answer two or three times (For example: "I wish I had better communication with my father.") The same is done for "I want . . ." and "I am . . ."

Important: Try to be positive with your language. (For example, instead of "I am a binger," say, "I am curing myself of binge eating.")

4. **Discussion:** This meeting's topic is "Family Relations." Each group member takes three uninterrupted minutes to describe their family. It may be helpful to address how your family relates, your parents' and siblings' characters, and the atmosphere at family get-togethers. After everyone has had a chance to speak, open the floor to discussion and questions. Listen carefully! Try to understand some of the reasons for your eating behavior.

5. **Exercise:** Assertiveness to Mom or Dad!

For the first part of this exercise, everyone writes some things that they *dislike* about one parent (living or dead, past or present). Then, take turns sharing answers, and continue until everyone has spoken two or three times. Go around again stressing their *likable* traits. Continue this until everyone has spoken at least three times. (Example: "I dislike how financially dependent my mother acts," and "I like that my mom listens when I talk to her.")

The second part of this exercise is a gripe session with mother or father. Get in pairs or triads and take turns spending about ten minutes in role-playing that allows you to assert yourself to your parent(s). You may bring up old wounds that have never healed, you may scream, or you may try to explain your feelings. Express your true self in a way that you have always wished you could. Even though this is only a role-play, try to be serious and avoid hiding your feelings. When playing the parent role, try to put yourself fully into that person's character.

6. **Relaxation:** Take five minutes for group relaxation, led by a volunteer. This can be as simple sitting quietly with your eyes closed, repeating an affirmation, or using another technique described in this book.

7. Set a time and place for the next meeting.

8. Share a few words about commitment to the group. Dis-

cuss if any members want to rely on each other for support outside of the meetings.

Note: Do not procrastinate working on your individual steps towards getting better. If you need to seek professional therapy, have a medical examination, tell more people about your bulimia, or whatever—*do it!*

Third Meeting Agenda

1. If appropriate, appoint a new facilitator, time-keeper, and gripe-control monitor.

2. Review the guidelines of the group and agenda.

3. **Introduction:** Each person spends a few minutes sharing a success story about how they stopped themselves from bingeing. If you don't have a success story, say so, and suggest something you might try to do instead of bingeing in the future. It's important to be honest!

4. **Discussion:** This meeting's topics are "rituals" and "secrecy." Most bulimics are secretive about their food obsessions and engage in private rituals involving scales, mirrors, clothing, or food. They may even compulsively lie and steal. Each person reveals some of their secrets and answers questions. (For example: "Every time I close the bathroom door, I automatically check myself in the mirror," or "I shoplift cosmetics.") Disclosing secrets takes away some of the importance and power you have given them.

5. **Exercise:** Visualization

Repeat the progressive relaxation technique from the first meeting. Then, the narrator tells the group to imagine themselves in front of a mirror, and to think about how they would look as a different race, a child, an old person, very ugly, the opposite sex, fat, thin, very beautiful, and finally, as light without form. (The narrator might suggest these possibilities one at a time, pausing for reflection before continuing to the next description.) Then, instruct the group to visualize themselves stepping through the mirror and feeling absorbed by that light, filled with health, purity, love, and contentment. Remain in this state for a few minutes before slowly reviving.

6. **Summary:** Discuss the effectiveness of the group. How can it be improved? What are everyone's feelings about the group? Are people willing to commit to attend through the next three guided meetings? Does the group then want to: continue, disband, enlist a therapist (if there is not one already), etc. Start making plans now.

7. Set a time and place for the next meeting.

Fourth Meeting Agenda

1. If appropriate, appoint a new facilitator, time-keeper, and gripe-control monitor.

2. Review the guidelines and agenda.

3. **Introduction:** Each person shares a brief story about a positive step towards their recovery they have taken or experienced since starting the support group. This may be an action, thought, or feeling.

4. **Discussion:** "The Media, Feminism, and Food."

This is an open-ended discussion. Try to keep comments related to personal experiences. Consider these questions:

- Why are bulimics mainly women?
- How does the media affect your body image?

- Why is there competition between women over their appearance? Does it have to be this way?
- What role do men play in perpetuating negative stereotypes about women?

5. **Exercise:** Equality

Every person takes turns bringing up positive and negative characterizations of women on television shows. Point out stereotypes that promote thinness as desireable, fat women as unappealing, and good role models. How would the shows be different if these actresses reversed roles?

6. **Discuss the future of the group.** There are still two more meeting agendas provided. What are everyone's feelings about the group? Are people willing to attend those guided meetings? What direction is the group going to take? Is the group open to new members? A decision should be reached by the next meeting. Set a time and place.

7. **Close with some suggestions:** What can we do as individuals on a daily basis to improve our self-image?

Fifth Meeting Agenda

1. If appropriate, appoint a new facilitator, time-keeper, and gripe-control monitor.

2. Review the guidelines and agenda.

3. **Introduction:** Each person shares a positive experience with self-help ideas or professional therapy.

4. **Discussion:** "Feelings are not good or bad, they just are."

Bulimics are often "people pleasers" who tend to keep their real feelings hidden. They are said to "swallow their feelings" instead of being honest about them. To get this discussion started, take turns naming types of feelings (happiness, fear, excitement, etc.). Then, discuss the following topics or others that develop.

- How can we identify feelings as they happen rather than hiding from them?
- What are different ways of coping with difficult feelings?
- What is so scary about expressing feelings?

5. **Exercise:** The Bulimic Cycle.

Bulimics follow a pattern of feelings and behaviors that make up the binge/purge cycle. Sit a circle taking turns describing consecutive parts of the cycle. For example: "I feel anxious," might be followed by "I start thinking about food," all the way until, "I throw up," and "I feel guilty." Go into as much detail as the individuals want, and keep going until the cycle starts to be replayed. When you reach this point, the next person should interrupt the bulimic cycle by saying, "I recognize I must do something else instead of bingeing." Then, take turns with suggestions for how to proceed in a healthier direction.

6. **Summary:** Resolve the group's future. This is a good time to consider inviting a trained therapist to the next meeting, if that has not already been done.

7. Set a time and place for the next meeting.

8. Share your feelings about the group's effectiveness.

Sixth Meeting Agenda

1. Appoint a new facilitator, time-keeper, and gripe-control monitor.

2. Review the agenda.

3. **Introduction:** In what positive ways have you changed since joining the group? New members can answer the intro-

ductory questions from the first meeting's agenda. Everyone takes a turn.

4. **The Future of the Group:** If your group's future is uncertain at this time, make it a top priority. Spend as much time as needed to finish up this matter. Work together to develop discussion topics and exercises if there are going to be more meetings. You might find some good ideas in Chapter Nine of this book.

5. **Discussion:** Intimacy

Most bulimics have withdrawn from normal social interaction and lost touch with what it means to be in open, mutually rewarding relationships. They are afraid to express opinions and feel that they might inconvenience others with their needs. They think everyone disapproves of them. Take turns answering the following questions, and discuss the answers:

- What good qualities can you bring to a friendship?
- What kind of first impression do you think you make?
- Is there anyone with whom you can be completely yourself?
- Do you want to get closer to any group members in or out of meetings?

6. **Exercise:** Feeling Connected

Everyone gets in a circle and holds hands. One person squeezes their left hand (their partner's right), and the squeeze is passed around the circle from person to person. At random, reverse the direction. Continue this playful exchange for a couple of minutes. Then, while still remaining connected, take turns thanking the group and members for their support.

Resources

Non-Profit Associations

AED
Academy for Eating Disorders
Degnon Associates, Inc.
6728 Old McLean Village Dr.
McLean, VA 22101-3906
(703) 556-9222
www.acadeatdis.org
For eating disorders professionals; promotes effective treatment, develops prevention initiatives, stimulates research, sponsors international conference. Also gives referrals.

ANAD
National Association of Anorexia Nervosa and Associated Disorders
Box 7
Highland Park, IL 60035
(708)831-3438
www.healthtouch.com/level1/leaflets/anad/anad001.htm
Distributes listing of therapists, hospitals and informative materials; sponsors support groups, conference, research, and a crisis hot line.

EDAP
Eating Disorders Awareness and Prevention
603 Stewart St. #803
Seattle, WA 98101
(206) 382-3587
members.aol.com/edapinc/home.html
Sponsors Eating Disorders Awareness Week annually in February with a network of state coordinators and programs; distributes educational information, annual conference, and advocacy. Their referral and general info line is: (800) 931-2237.

IAEDP
International Association of Eating Disorders Professionals
427 Wooping Lop #1819
Alta Monte Springs, FL 32701
(800) 800-8126
www.iaedp.com
A membership organization for professionals; provides certification, education, local chapters, a newsletter, and an annual symposium. Also gives referrals.

NEDO
National Eating Disorders Organization
6655 S. Yale Ave.
Tulsa, OK 74136
(918) 481-4044
www.laureate.com/nedo-con.html
Focuses on prevention, education, research, and treatment referrals; distributes information.

Books and Internet

The Eating Disorders Resource Catalogue
PO Box 2238
Carlsbad, CA 92018
(800)756-7533
www.bulimia.com
Offers free catalogue of more than 125 books on eating disorders, non-profit associations, and treatment facilities. The Internet site includes books, links to many other eating disorders pages, lists of videos, with information about and links to treatment facilities.

Eating Disorders: A Reference Sourcebook
by Ray Lemberg, Ph.D. with Leigh Cohn
Oryx Press
4041 North Central at Indian School Rd.
Phoenix, AZ 85012
(602)265-6250
This book has current information about eating disorders and also includes an extensive bibliography, a list of videos, and addresses and descriptions of inpatient treatment programs.

The Eating Disorders Sourcebook
by Carolyn Costin, M.A., M.Ed. M.F.C.C.
Lowell House/NTC
4255 West Touhy Ave.
Lincolnwood, IL 60646
(800)323-4900
This book is a comprehensive guide to eating disorders, and includes a section with addresses and descriptions of many treatment programs.

The Gürze Books Eating Disorders Website
www.gurze.com
Includes more than 150 books on eating disorders and related topics with photos and annotations; video and audio tapes; links to treatment facilities, non-profit organizations, and other related information sites; *Eating Disorders Review* references; and e-mail to Lindsey Hall.

The Something Fishy Website on Eating Disorders
www.something-fishy.com
Signs and symptoms, physical dangers, definitions, words for victims sufferings, family and friends bulletin board, treatment options, a memorial page dedicated to people who have died of eating disorders, Links to other sites, chat rooms, guest speakers, and much more.

The Mirror-Mirror Website on Eating Disorders
www.mirror-mirror.org/eatdis.htm
Definitions, signs and symptoms, physical dangers, specific information on athletes, men and children with eating disorders, relapse warning signs, and much more; also has links to many web personal sites from individuals who have had or recovered from eating disorders.

Bibliography

American Psychiatric Association (APA). *Diagnostic and Statistical Manual of Mental Disorders (4th ed.).* Washington, DC: APA, 1994.

Andersen, Arnold. "Eating Disorders in Males: Critical Questions" in Lemberg, 1999.

Bock, Linda. "Differential Diagnoses, Co-Morbidities, and Complications of Eating Disorders" in Lemberg, 1999.

Buckroyd, Julia. *Anorexia and Bulimia: Your Questions Answered.* Shaftesbury, Dorset, UK: Element Books Limited, 1996.

Cavanaugh, Carolyn. and Lemberg, Raymond. "What We Know About Eating Disorders: Facts and Statistics" in Lemberg, 1999.

Chernin, Kim. *The Obsession: Reflections on the Tyranny of Slenderness.* New York: HarperCollins, 1981.

Collins, M. "Body Figure Perception and Preferences Among Preadolescent Children." *International Journal of Eating Disorders,* 10, 1991.

Costin, Carolyn. "Tending the Soul in Therapy." *Eating Disorders: The Journal of Treatment and Prevention,* 6:2; Summer, 1998.

Crisp, Arthur H., Joughin, N., Halek, C., et. al. *Anorexia Nervosa: The Wish to Change, Second Edition*. East Sussex, UK: Psychology Press, 1996.

Ellis-Ordway, Nancy. "Are You Really 'Too Fat'? The Role of Culture and Weight Stereotypes" in Lemberg, 1999.

Fallon, Patricia, Katzman, Melanie, and Wooley, Susan. *Feminist Perspectives on Eating Disorders*. New York: Guilford Press, 1994.

Fodor, Viola. *Desperately Seeking Self*. Carlsbad, CA: Gürze Books, 1997.

Foreyt, John and Goodrick, Ken. *Living Without Dieting*. New York: Warner Books, 1992.

Gaesser, Glenn. *Big Fat Lies*. New York: Random House, 1996.

Garfinkel, Paul and Walsh, B. Timothy. "Drug Therapies" in Garner, 1997.

Garner, David M. and Garfinkel, Paul E., eds. *Handbook of Treatment for Eating Disorders, Second Edition*. New York: Guilford Press, 1997.

Goodman, Charisse W. *The Invisible Woman: Confronting Weight Prejudice in America*. Carlsbad, CA: Gürze Books, 1995.

Hall, Lindsey with Cohn, Leigh. *Eat Without Fear: A True Story of the Binge-Purge Syndrome*. Santa Barbara, CA: Gürze Books, 1980.

Hall, Lindsey and Ostroff, Monika. *Anorexia Nervosa: A Guide To Recovery*. Carlsbad, CA: Gürze Books, 1998.

Johnson, Craig and Connors, Mary. *The Etiology and Treatment of Bulimia Nervosa*. New York: Basic Books, 1987.

Kaye, Walter and Strober, Michael. "Serotonin: Implications for the Etiology and Treatment of Eating Disorders." *Eating Disorders Review,* 10:3; May/June 1999.

Lemberg, Raymond. with Cohn, Leigh. *Eating Disorders: A Reference Sourcebook*. Phoenix, AZ: Oryx Press, 1999.

Mellin, L.M., Irwin, C.E., Scully, S. "Prevalence of Disordered Eating in Girls: A Survey of Middle-Class Children." *Journal of American Dietetic Association,* 92, (7), 1992

Mickley, Diane. "Medical Dangers of Anorexia Nervosa and Bulimia Nervosa" in Lemberg, 1999.

Mitchell, James, Specker, Sheila, and Edmonson, Karen. "Management of Substance Abuse and Dependence" in Garner, 1997.

Piran, Niva. "Prevention of Eating Disorders: The Struggle to Chart New Territories." *Eating Disorders: The Journal of Treatment and Prevention,* 6:4; Winter, 1998.

Russell, Gerald. "The History of Bulimia Nervosa" in Garner, 1997.

Sandbeck, Terence. *The Deadly Diet: Recovering from Anorexia and Bulimia*. Oakland, CA: New Harbinger Publications, 1993.

Schwartz, Mark and Cohn, Leigh. *Sexual Abuse and Eating Disorders*. New York: Brunner/Mazel, 1996.

Seid, Roberta. "Too 'Close to the Bone': The Historical Context for Women's Obsession with Slenderness" in Fallon, 1994.

Siegel, Michele; Brisman, Judith; and Weinshel, Margot. *Surviving an Eating Disorder: Strategies for Family and Friends*. New York: HarperCollins, 1997

Vanderlinden, Johan and Vandereycken, Walter. "Is Sexual Abuse a Risk Factor for Developing an Eating Disorder?" in Schwartz, 1996.

Yager, Joel, ed. "Postpartum Period: A Time of Increased Concern about Weight and Shape." *Eating Disorders Review 8:4,* 1997.

Zerbe, Kathryn. *The Body Betrayed: A Deeper Understanding of Women, Eating Disorders, and Treatment*. Carlsbad, CA: Gürze Books, 1995.

Index

About the Authors

Lindsey Hall and **Leigh Cohn** are married and the authors of several books on eating disorders and recovery topics. Among their best-known titles are *Anorexia Nervosa: A Guide to Recovery* (Lindsey and Monika Ostroff), *Self-Esteem Tools for Recovery,* and *Full Lives: Women Who Have Freed Themselves from Food & Weight Obsession,* all of which have been translated into other languages, such as French, Italian, Japanese, and Chinese. Their company, Gürze Books, publishes books related to eating disorders by a wide array of respected authors.

Lindsey is a graduate of Stanford University with a B.A. in Psychology (1971) and was the first recovered bulimic to appear on national television to share her story. She served as Executive Director of Eating Disorders Awareness and Prevention, Inc. and in the late '70s pioneered the soft-sculpture art form, designing and selling more than a half-million Gürze dolls throughout the world. Leigh, who has an M.A.T. from Northwestern University (1975) is Executive Editor of *Eating Disorders: The Journal of Treatment and Prevention,* a peer review newsletter for clinicians, and is a past president of Publishers Marketing Association. Lindsey and Leigh are the parents of two sons, Neil and Charlie.

About the Publisher

Since 1980, Gürze Books has specialized in quality information on eating disorders recovery, research, education, advocacy, and prevention. The company distributes *The Eating Disorders Resource Catalogue,* which is used as a resource throughout the world, and publishes the *Eating Disorders Review,* a newsletter for professionals. The Gürze Books website (www.bulimia.com) is an excellent resource and Internet gateway to treatment facilities, associations, and other eating disorders sites.

Also Available by Lindsey Hall

FREE Eating Disorders Resource Catalogue

This widely-used resource has more than 125 books on eating disorders and related topics, listings of non-profit association and treatment facilities, and basic facts. It is handed out by therapists, educators, and other health care professionals.

Understanding Bulimia by Lindsey Hall

(55 min. audio tape) $10.00

This 1983 recording provides a revealing look at this secretive food obsession. Hall candidly describes how a seemingly innocent diet became a nine-year addiction, how the bulimic behavior became a substitute for relationships, her feelings about bingeing and vomiting, and how she recovered.

The Bulimia Coat by Lindsey Hall

(60 min. audio tape) $10.00

Recorded in 1991 at an eating disorders conference in Colorado Springs, this tape is an inspirational talk by Hall on the relationship between bulimia, self-esteem, and love. She talks about how bulimia is a form of protection, like a "coat," that must be taken off gradually and gently. She also shares the rewards of her own recovery—feelings of happiness, spiritual contentment, and total freedom from food and weight concerns.

Anorexia Nervosa: A Guide to Recovery

by Lindsey Hall & Monika Ostroff $13.95   1998

Using the same basic format as *Bulimia: A Guide to Recovery*, this guidebook for understanding and overcoming anorexia nervosa includes answers to commonly asked questions; Monika's own story of abuse, self-starvation, and recovery; specific things to do that have worked for others in recovery; information on healthy eating and weight; suggestions for how to stay committed; and a special section for parents and loved ones.

Self-Esteem Tools for Recovery

by Lindsey Hall & Leigh Cohn $10.95   1990

Hall and Cohn wrote this book to help readers experience their innermost selves, the source of true self-esteem. It speaks directly to people who have decided that their coping mechanisms no longer serve them as lifestyles. Included are short, specific tools, easy-to-use exercises, and pertinent examples to help readers gain confidence in making decisions, make peace with the past, overcome destructive thoughts and behavior, and live in a state of love and compassion.

Full Lives: Women Who Have Freed Themselves from Food and Weight Obsession

by Lindsey Hall $13.95   1993

In this entertaining book, Hall introduces 16 extraordinary women who have overcome food and weight obsessions, as though they are all dining together at a large circular table, taking turns talking about themselves and the lessons they've learned from food. Their personal transformation are for all readers who need encouragement to lead a full life of their own.

Order Form

_____ **FREE** copies of the *Eating Disorders Bookshelf Catalogue*

_____ Copies of *Bulimia: A Guide to Recovery - Fifth Edition*
$14.95 each - 5 or more copies @ $11.95

_____ Copies of *Understanding Bulimia (55 min. audio tape)*
$10.00 each - 5 or more copies @ $8.00

_____ Copies of *The Bulimia Coat (60 min. audio tape)*
$10.00 each - 5 or more copies @ $8.00

_____ Copies of *Anorexia Nervosa: A Guide to Recovery*
$13.95 each - 5 or more copies @ $10.95

_____ Copies of *Self-Esteem Tools for Recovery*
$10.95 each - 5 or more copies @ $8.50

_____ Copies of *Full Lives: Women Who Have Freed Themselves
from Food & Weight Obsessions*
$13.95 each - 5 or more copies @ $10.95

Shipping & Handling for books & tapes:
One item @ $3.00, 2-9 copies @ $2.00 ea., 10+ copies @ $1.65 each

California residents add 7.75% sales tax.
Pay by check, Mastercard, Visa, or American Express.

NAME _____

ADDRESS _____

CITY/ST/ZIP _____

PHONE _____

Gürze Books (B5) • P.O. Box 2238 • Carlsbad, CA 92018
(800)756-7533 • (760)434-7533 • www.bulimia.com